D0417474

my
YOGA
guru
Your ultimate yoga instructor

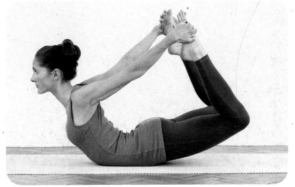

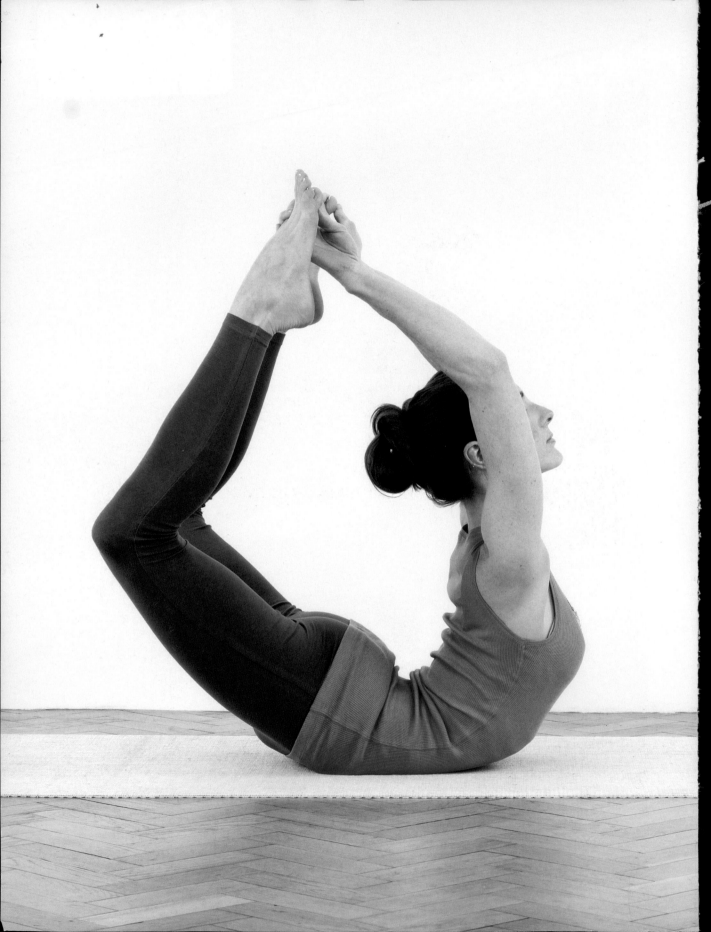

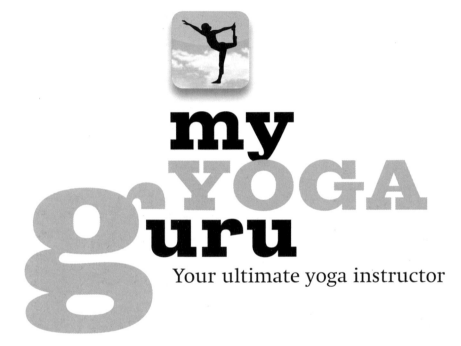

my YOGA guru

Your ultimate yoga instructor

DORY WALKER

hamlyn

An Hachette UK Company

www.hachette.co.uk

First published in Great Britain in 2012 by
Hamlyn, a division of Octopus Publishing Group Ltd
Endeavour House
189 Shaftesbury Avenue
London
WC2H 8JY

www.octopusbooks.co.uk

ISBN 9780600622307

A CIP catalogue record for this book is available from the
British Library

Printed and bound in China

10 9 8 7 6 5 4 3 2 1

Disclaimer
Any information given in this book is not intended to be taken
as a replacement for medical advice. Any person with a
condition requiring medical attention should consult a
qualified medical practitioner or therapist before beginning
any of the postures in this book. Whilst the advice and
information in this book is believed to be accurate and the
advice, instruction, or formulae have been devised to avoid
strain, neither the author nor the publisher will be responsible
for any injury, losses, damages, actions, proceedings, claims,
demands, expenses and costs (including legal costs or
expenses) incurred or any way arising out of following the
exercises in this book.

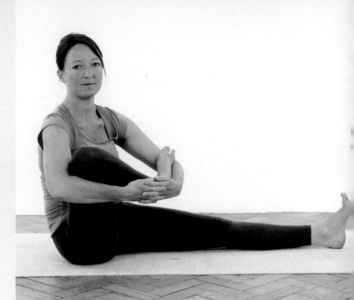

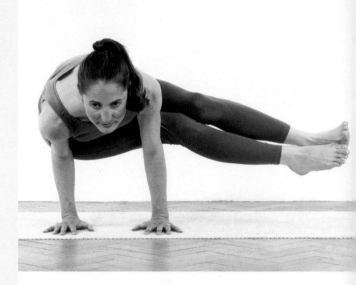

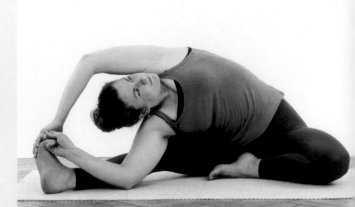

Contents

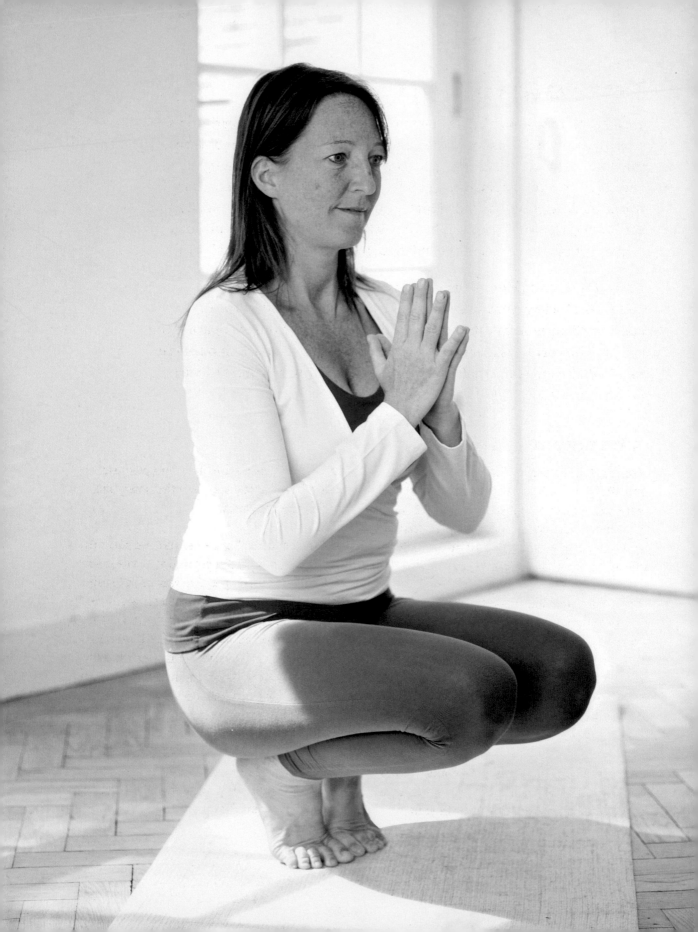

Introduction

Yoga has so much to offer. It is an in-depth, scientific system with roots that can be traced back more than 10,000 years. It is ancient and sacred, said to be of revealed knowledge, a gift to humanity from the wise yogis and sages of yore. Originating in India, yoga is a complete system that works on developing the individual, physically, mentally, emotionally and spiritually. The word yoga can be translated as 'union' and the ultimate goal of yoga is the union of the individual Self with the universal Self.

It has relevance now more than ever. With high levels of stress in a materialist society, yoga strengthens the mind to control desires and cultivate discernment. Whatever age you are, wherever you come from, you can practise yoga. It is a universal discipline that has relevance and benefit for all. It also offers the tools to live pain-free in our bodies and fosters a positive mental outlook.

The power of yoga

This book is an easy-to-follow introduction into classical hatha yoga practices together with some simple meditation techniques. It is a guide to get you started and then inspire you to go deeper into this vast and hugely rewarding path of self-discovery.

The main thing about yoga is practice. No one can really tell you what it is like, you have to experience it for yourself to see and experience the benefits, which are immense. It is a mighty subject and, as such, needs to be approached with humility and an open heart. It is about us, the stuff we are made of, the elements and how they work together.

Through yoga you can learn to connect to the fire in your belly, the ground at your feet, the air in your breath and the ether in your thoughts. There is a history and purpose behind all the poses, connecting everyone to the natural world.

Yoga is a spiritual practice, and the poses in this book are just the beginning to open you to an effective and positive way of living in every moment. Start by gaining more of an understanding about yoga on pages 12–19, then read about the basic, but essential, practices of breathing and relaxation. It is then time to move into the postures themselves, which start with those for beginners and move through to the most advanced. In hatha yoga, meditation is just as important an element as the postures, so it is explained on pages 144–53 before a choice of detailed yoga sessions. Yoga provides a complete philosophy for living; *My Yoga Guru* leads the way on the beginning of that journey.

How to use My Yoga Guru

My Yoga Guru is an easy-to-use, meticulously structured guide to the world of yoga. Taking you from the basics through to advanced poses and ending with specifically designed sessions, each element aims to ensure you are equipped with maximum knowledge for best practice.

Introducing My Yoga Guru

About yoga (see pages 12–19) explains the different aspects of yoga and which parts are focused on in this book.

Basic practices (see pages 20–33) explain core techniques, including breathing and relaxing (see below).

Three further chapters of postures – beginner (see pages 34–59), intermediate (see pages 60–111) and advanced (see pages 112–43) – explore yoga poses from the simplest to the most strenuous. You are always led by the hand to maximize your potential (see opposite, top).

Meditation (see pages 144–53) is an important element of yoga. This chapter explains its ethos and how to do it.

Yoga sessions (see pages 152–73) designed for you to explore in different ways (see opposite, bottom) round off the book.

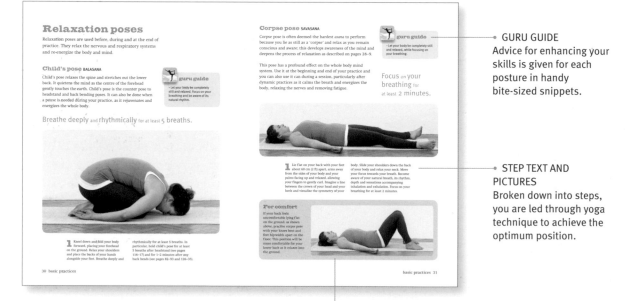

GURU GUIDE
Advice for enhancing your skills is given for each posture in handy bite-sized snippets.

STEP TEXT AND PICTURES
Broken down into steps, you are led through yoga technique to achieve the optimum position.

Starting off

The first two chapters set the scene. Revisit them frequently to remind yourself how to get the most from the poses described in subsequent chapters.

ALTERNATIVE PICTURES
Extra information is provided to help you with greater comfort or better positioning.

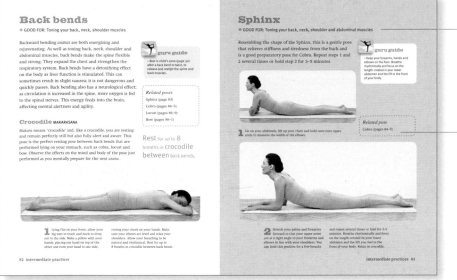

Back bends

◆ GOOD FOR: Toning your back, neck, shoulder muscles

Backward bending asanas are both energizing and rejuvenating. As well as toning back, neck, shoulder and abdominal muscles, back bends make the spine flexible and strong. They expand the chest and strengthen the respiratory system. Back bends have a detoxifying effect on the body as liver function is stimulated. This can sometimes result in slight nausea; it is not dangerous and quickly passes. Back bending also has a neurological effect; as circulation is increased in the spine, more oxygen is fed to the spinal nerves. This energy feeds into the brain, affecting mental alertness and agility.

Crocodile MAKARASANA

Makara means 'crocodile' and, like a crocodile, you are resting and remain perfectly still but also fully alert and aware. This pose is the perfect resting pose between back bends that are performed lying on your stomach, such as cobra, locust and bow. Observe the effects on the mind and body of the pose just performed as you mentally prepare for the next asana.

guru guide
• Rest in child's pose (page 30) after a back bend or twist, to release and realign the spine and back muscles.

Related poses
Sphinx (page 83)
Cobra (pages 84–5)
Locust (pages 86–9)
Bow (pages 90–1)

Rest for up to 8 breaths in crocodile between back bends.

1 Lying flat on your front, allow your big toes to touch and heels to drop out to the side. Make a pillow with your hands, placing one hand on top of the other and turn your head to one side. resting your cheek on your hands. Make sure your elbows are level and relax your hands. Allow your breathing to be natural and rhythmical. Rest for up to 8 breaths in crocodile between back bends.

82 intermediate practices

Sphinx

◆ GOOD FOR: Toning your back, neck, shoulder and abdominal muscles

Resembling the shape of the Sphinx, this is a gentle pose that relieves stiffness and tiredness from the back and is a good preparatory pose for Cobra. Repeat steps 1 and 2 several times or hold step 2 for 3–5 minutes.

guru guide
• Keep your forearms, hands and elbows on the floor. Breathe rhythmically and focus on the length created in your lower abdomen and the lift in the front of your body.

1 Lie on your abdomen, lift up your chest and hold onto your upper arms to measure the width of the elbows.

Related pose
Cobra (pages 84–5)

2 Stretch your palms and forearms forward so that your upper arms are at a right angle to your forearms and elbows in line with your shoulders. You can hold this position for a few breaths and repeat several times or hold for 3–5 minutes. Breathe rhythmically and focus on the length created in your lower abdomen and the lift you feel in the front of your body. Relax in crocodile.

intermediate practices 83

• GOOD FOR
This information explains the core purpose of each posture.

• RELATED POSES
Many yoga poses are related to each other. To help you find your way around the book, page numbers are given for relevant postures.

Yoga practices

Each aspect of yoga technique is carefully explained for every posture. They are ordered sequentially within appropriately levelled chapters, as for a yoga sequence.

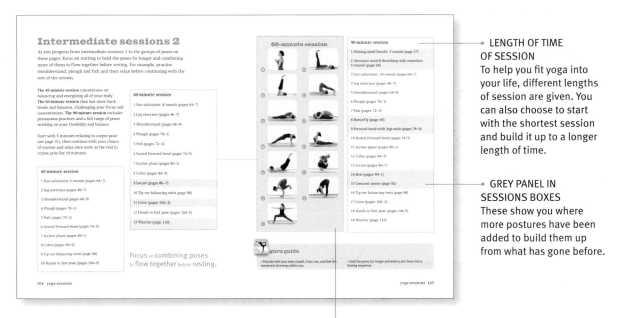

Intermediate sessions 2

As you progress from intermediate sessions 1 to the groups of poses on these pages, focus on starting to hold the poses for longer and combining more of them to flow together before resting. For example, practise shoulderstand, plough and fish and then relax before continuing with the rest of the session.

The 45-minute session concentrates on balancing and energizing all of your body. **The 60-minute session** then has more back bends and balances, challenging your focus and concentration. **The 90-minute session** includes pranayama practices and a full range of poses working on your flexibility and balance.

Start with 5 minutes relaxing in corpse pose (see page 31), then continue with your choice of routine and relax once more at the end in corpse pose for 10 minutes.

45-minute session
1 Sun salutation: 6 rounds (pages 64–7)
2 Leg exercises (pages 46–7)
3 Shoulderstand (pages 68–9)
4 Plough (pages 70–1)
5 Fish (pages 72–3)
6 Seated forward bend (pages 74–5)
7 Incline plane (pages 80–1)
8 Cobra (pages 84–5)
9 Tip toe balancing twist (page 98)
10 Hands to feet pose (pages 104–5)

60-minute session
1 Sun salutation: 8 rounds (pages 64–7)
2 Leg exercises (pages 46–7)
3 Shoulderstand (pages 68–9)
4 Plough (pages 70–1)
5 Fish (pages 72–3)
6 Seated forward bend (pages 74–5)
7 Incline plane (pages 80–1)
8 Cobra (pages 84–5)
9 Locust (pages 86–7)
10 Tip toe balancing twist (page 98)
11 Crow (pages 102–3)
12 Hands to feet pose (pages 104–5)
13 Warrior (page 110)

Focus on combining poses to flow together before resting.

60-minute session

90-minute session
1 Shining skull breath: 3 rounds (page 27)
2 Alternate nostril breathing with retention: 5 rounds (page 26)
3 Sun salutation: 10 rounds (pages 64–7)
4 Leg exercises (pages 46–7)
5 Shoulderstand (pages 68–9)
6 Plough (pages 70–1)
7 Fish (pages 72–3)
8 Butterfly (page 45)
9 Forward bend with legs wide (pages 78–9)
10 Seated forward bend (pages 74–5)
11 Incline plane (pages 80–1)
12 Cobra (pages 84–5)
13 Locust (pages 86–7)
14 Bow (pages 90–1)
15 Crescent moon (page 92)
16 Tip toe balancing twist (page 98)
17 Crow (pages 102–3)
18 Hands to feet pose (pages 104–5)
19 Warrior (page 110)

guru guide
• Practise with your eyes closed, if you can, and feel the movement of energy within you.
• Hold the poses for longer and work to join them into a flowing sequence.

164 yoga sessions

yoga sessions 165

• LENGTH OF TIME OF SESSION
To help you fit yoga into your life, different lengths of session are given. You can also choose to start with the shortest session and build it up to a longer length of time.

• GREY PANEL IN SESSIONS BOXES
These show you where more postures have been added to build them up from what has gone before.

Yoga sessions

Carefully crafted sessions divided into beginner, intermediate and advanced levels, and to various lengths of time, are given on pages 158–73.

• PHOTO PANEL
Pictures for each posture in one routine (here, for the 60-minute session) act as a memory aid.

Your free App

My Yoga Guru is designed to be a complete package. It comes with a free iPhone application that is downloadable from iTunes. With this application you will be able to:

- View poses.
- Create your own yoga sessions.
- View pre-loaded or saved sessions.
- Monitor your progress and record your development.

Downloading the App

To download the App, simply go to the App Store and type in 'My Yoga Guru'. The App you want has the 'My Guru' logo (right).

Note: you can download the application for either iPhone or iPad and it is compatible with any version.

The App is simple to use and follow. After the title screen you will be given a number of options:

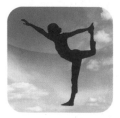

My Yoga Guru

1. Introduction

This explains how best to use the application and point those with just the App towards the book for the complete My Guru package.

2. Explore exercises

Here you can view all the exercises in the book together with their variations. You can search the exercises in different ways:

- Those that are good for a particular thing, such as flexibility or joints.
- Skill level: beginner, intermediate or advanced.
- Those you've marked as favourite.
- By keyword.

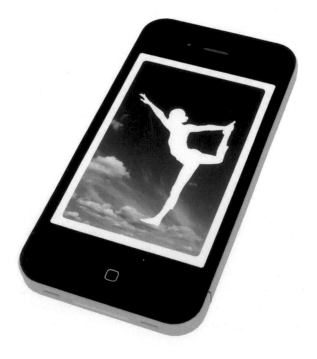

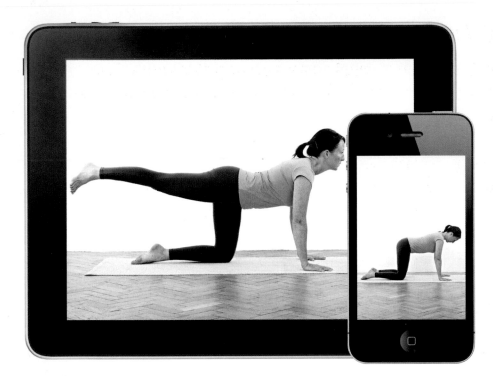

Each individual pose screen shows you what skill level the position is and what it's good for. It also has options to add the pose to a session, mark it as a favourite and share the fact you're doing it on social media.

Tapping on the image will allow you to see photographs of the steps of that exercise. These images are intended as a memory aid. Always refer to the book should you want specific step-by-step instruction.

3. Sessions

This is where you can build your own yoga sessions, save them, or follow the samples at the back of this book (see pages 154–173). All the yoga sessions from the book are here, so you've no need to build them yourself. The 'My sessions' tab will allow you to bring up the saved sessions, adapt them and rename them should you require.

For more advice about how to best structure your yoga sessions, refer to pages 156–157. Don't forget to hit the 'I've done this session' button at the end of every session so that your activity is recorded.

4. My results

This part of the App records the sessions you've completed so that you can monitor your progress over time by level and what the exercises are good for. You can also see which exercises and sessions you use the most and even monitor your weight and body mass index over time. This is an excellent way to see the benefits of your My Guru experience as your skills develop.

5. About My Gurus

This section gives you updated information about the latest books and packages in the series.

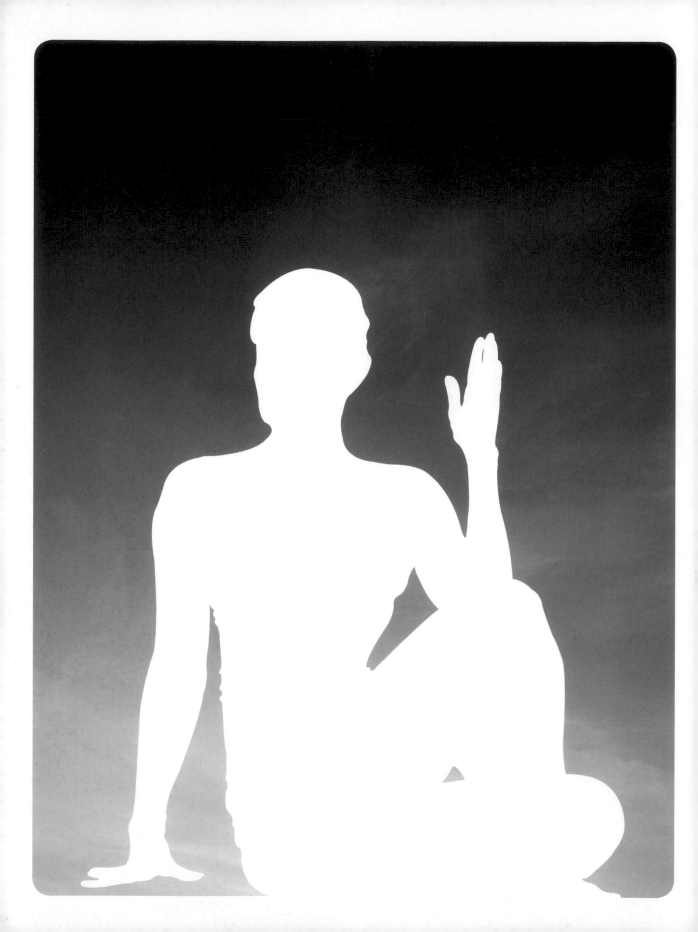

About Yoga

Yoga can be practised by everyone. It is an ancient discipline that connects mind, body and spirit. It is a system of positive living and is intended to be part of daily life. It allows us to step outside ourselves and explore our boundaries and, at the same time, takes us deep into our own hearts. It is a means to find harmony with yourself, with others and the environment. The key to success is committed practice, selfless service and study.

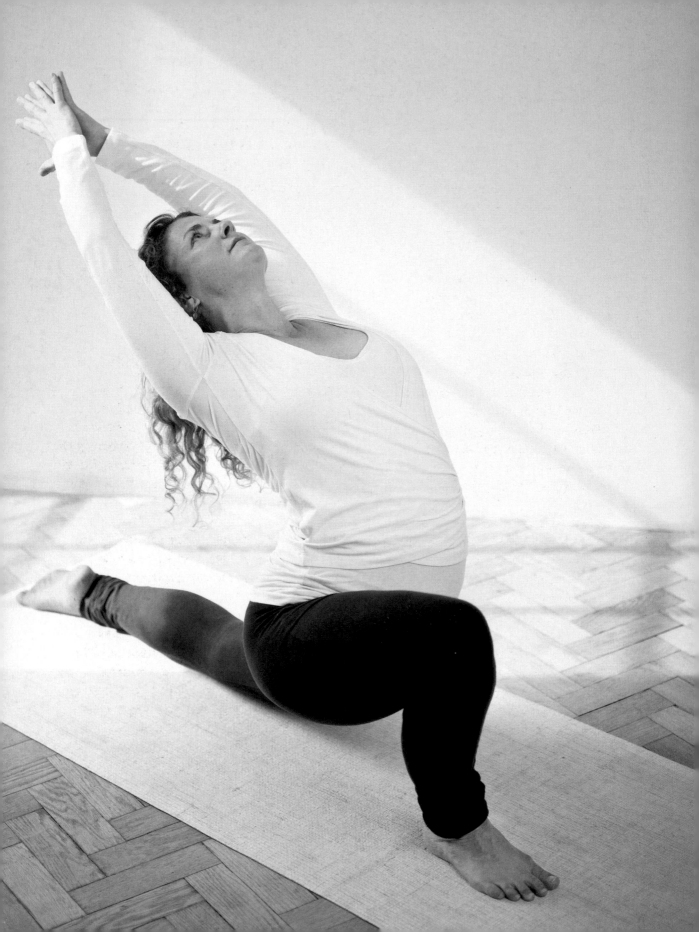

Understanding yoga

There are four paths that make up the complete system of yoga. These are raja, bhakti, karma and jnana yoga, translated as the yoga of the mind, the yoga of devotion, the yoga of action and the yoga of knowledge. Of these four paths, it is elements of raja yoga – the yoga of the mind – that are most widely practised in the West.

Raja yoga

This yogic path is an eight-limbed system that offers complete mastery of the mind. The eight steps of raja yoga are:

> *Yamas:* constraints
> *Niyamas:* observances
> *Asanas:* postures (proper exercise)
> *Pranayama:* breathing
> *Pratyahara:* withdrawal of the senses
> *Dharana:* concentration
> *Dhyana:* meditation
> *Samadhi:* super consciousness

The third and fourth steps in raja yoga – the *asanas* and *pranayama* – are those that are most commonly practised in the West and together they form hatha yoga (see pages 16–17). This is the area this book focuses on together with some simple meditation techniques.

The yamas and niyamas of raja yoga are guidelines for developing control of the senses and how you can live a moral life. They prepare the way to success in the practice of *asanas* and *pranayama*.

Pratyahara means drawing the senses in, shining the light of awareness inside. It is preparation for *dharana* concentration. Complete concentration involves being fully focused on one point, which leads naturally onto meditation or *dhyana*, and so onto *samadhi*, or super consciousness, the ultimate aim of yoga.

The other three paths

Bhakti yoga, the yoga of devotion, is a dedication of all actions as worship of the Divine. Chanting or singing God's name forms a substantial part of bhakti yoga. Inspired by the power of love, a bhakti practitioner transforms emotions into unconditional love and devotion through prayer and worship.

Karma yoga, the yoga of action, fosters the spirit of service in action. It is a means of purifying the heart by serving others.

Jnana yoga, the yoga of knowledge, is said to be the hardest path to follow. The jnana yogi uses his mind to delve into understanding the true reality of existence, his apparent separation from his true self and God. Through the use of his intellect the jnana yogi breaks down this false understanding and has direct experience of his unity with the Divine.

All four paths need to be integrated for an authentic yoga practice, but *asanas* and *pranayama* alone offer many benefits and often naturally lead the way along the other paths.

Hatha yoga

Hatha yoga is just one aspect of raja yoga, described on page 15. The main components of hatha yoga are *asanas* and *pranayama*, or the postures and breathing, and it is the part of yoga that most people think of when they hear the word yoga. Classical hatha yoga is a balancing system, the word *ha* meaning 'sun', and *tha*, the 'moon'. Hatha yoga, as taught in *The Hatha Yoga Pradipika* (see opposite), works on balancing the sun and moon energies that are within the microcosm of every human being.

Yogic science teaches that there are three bodies in man: the physical body, the astral and the causal. *Prana* is the energy that links the astral and physical bodies through channels known as *nadis. Sushumna nadi* is of greatest importance and can be likened to the spinal cord in the physical body, and *ida nadi* and *pingala nadi* start at the base of the spine, spiralling up and around *sushumna. Ida* carries the moon energy, or cooling energy, while *pingala* is the sun or heating energy.

Putting hatha yoga into practice

Hatha yoga is an integral system that balances the natural energies within our bodies.

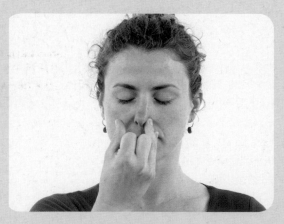

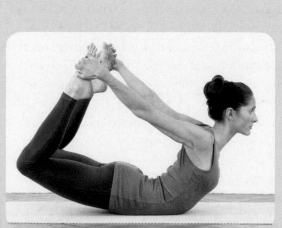

Anuloma viloma pranayama (see page 26) uses the energies of *ida nadi* and *pingala nadi* to balance the flow of breath and latent energy in the body.

The symmetry of a pose to equally extend, flex or compress a particular part of the body, such as the bow (see pages 90–1), works to balance the basic energy matrix that we hold.

Going back to its roots

Of the extensive literature written on yoga philosophy, the two main books relating to hatha yoga are *The Yoga Sutras of Patanjali*, which is the primary text on raja yoga, and *The Hatha Yoga Pradipika*. Classical yogic texts were mainly written in Sanskrit as the language's concise and poetic form lends itself well to spiritual instructions and philosophical discourse.

The literal meaning of sutra is 'thread'. As the sage Patanjali taught his students they noted down the essence of his teachings in short sentences, or groups of words – *sutras* that together weave the teachings of the science of yoga. As a result, *The Yoga Sutras of Patanjali* clearly sets down the aims and practices of yoga, the obstacles you may encounter on the path and how to remove them, and the precise results to be secured from the practices.

The other main manual on hatha yoga practices is *The Hatha Yoga Pradipika*, purportedly written down by Swatmarama yogi. It is a concise manual on hatha yoga, including *asanas*, *pranayama* and yoga philosophy. Written in the 15th century, it is said to be the oldest text on hatha yoga and retains its relevance to this day. The text is dedicated to Lord Shiva, one of the three main Hindu deities, the founder of yoga who is believed to have revealed the secrets of hatha yoga to his consort Parvati.

The practices presented in this book are classical hatha yoga, timeless in effectiveness and relevance. The tools to get you started and build and develop your own practice are provided here. It can in no way, however, be a substitute for a teacher as initiation on to the yogic path and for the spiritual transmission of knowledge.

Classical poses

These are some of the best-known classical poses that have been used in hatha yoga for centuries. Each one works on a different part of the body, resulting in an integral stretching and strengthening of the whole body.

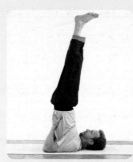

Sarvangasana – shoulder-stand (pages 68–9)

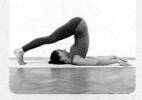

Halasana – plough (pages 70–1)

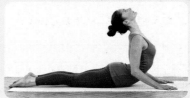

Bhujangasana – cobra (pages 84–5)

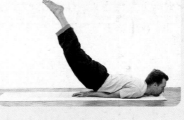

Salabhasana – locust (pages 86–7)

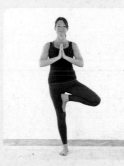

Vrksasana – tree (pages 100–1)

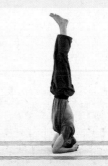

Sirasana – headstand (pages 116–17)

Yoga and health

Eat a little, drink a little,
Talk a little, sleep a little,
Mix a little, move a little,
Serve a little, rest a little
Work a little, relax a little   SWAMI SIVANANDA

Yoga is an integrated system with the health of the body, mind and spirit given equal importance. Together, yogic practices work on the healthy functioning of body and mind as the essence of yoga is about balance. It is the middle path of regularity and consistency, not of extremes. It is about right living and the choices that we make in day-to-day life.

Yoga is so much more than *pranayama* (breathing practices) and *asanas* (poses) working on the physical body alone, for they also work on the subtler energies within us. As more freedom and space is created within the body, so too is it in the mind. Yoga is therefore about proper exercise, breathing, relaxation, a wholesome nutritious diet, positive thinking and meditation. It is about fostering non-violence, honesty, generosity, kindness, compassion and contentment. As such, the regular practice of yoga increases energy levels, fosters a balanced state of mind and reduces stress levels and fatigue. Yoga brings life to life. It is about positive everyday living.

The three gunas

From a yogic perspective, everything has three qualities – or *gunas* – which are *sattva* (purity), *rajas* (activity) and *tamas* (inertia). They encompass all actions and all existence. In unmanifested form, the qualities are in balance, but on taking form, one quality always dominates. Eating and other activities that you enjoy, such as reading or walking, can be seen within these qualities, of which *sattva* is the most important for creating a calming and nourishing lifestyle – a healthy lifestyle.

Sattvic foods are those in their most natural form, they include fruit and vegetables, whole grains, seeds, nuts and milk. Walking in nature and reading inspirational words and listening to uplifting music all have a positive effect.

So take time to enjoy the simple things in life. Watch the sun rise, enjoy eating an apple, preparing a meal. All of these simple things done with a pure heart and presence enrich your yoga practice both on and off the mat.

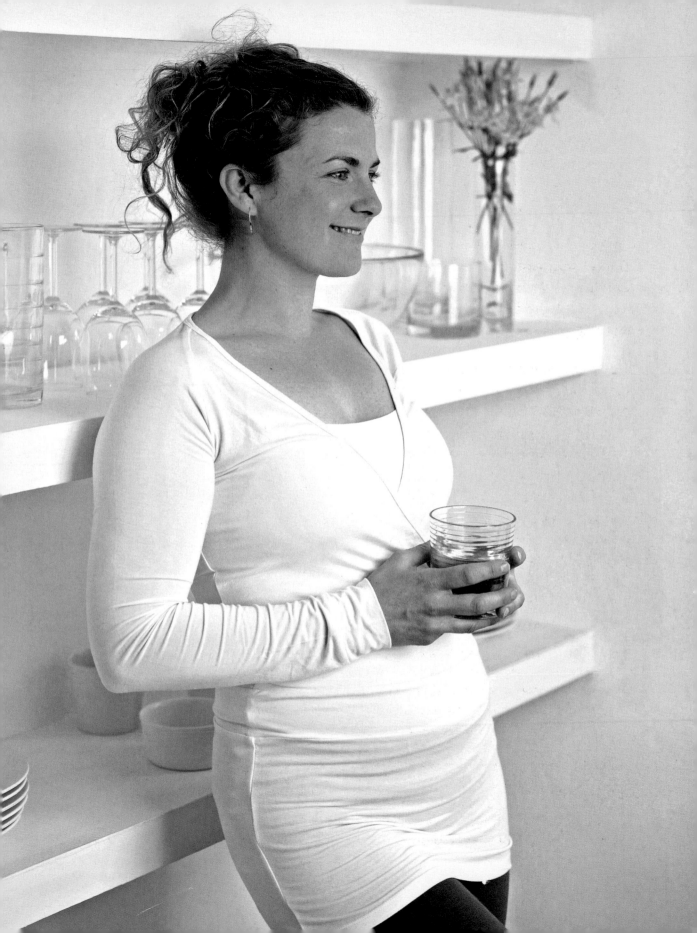

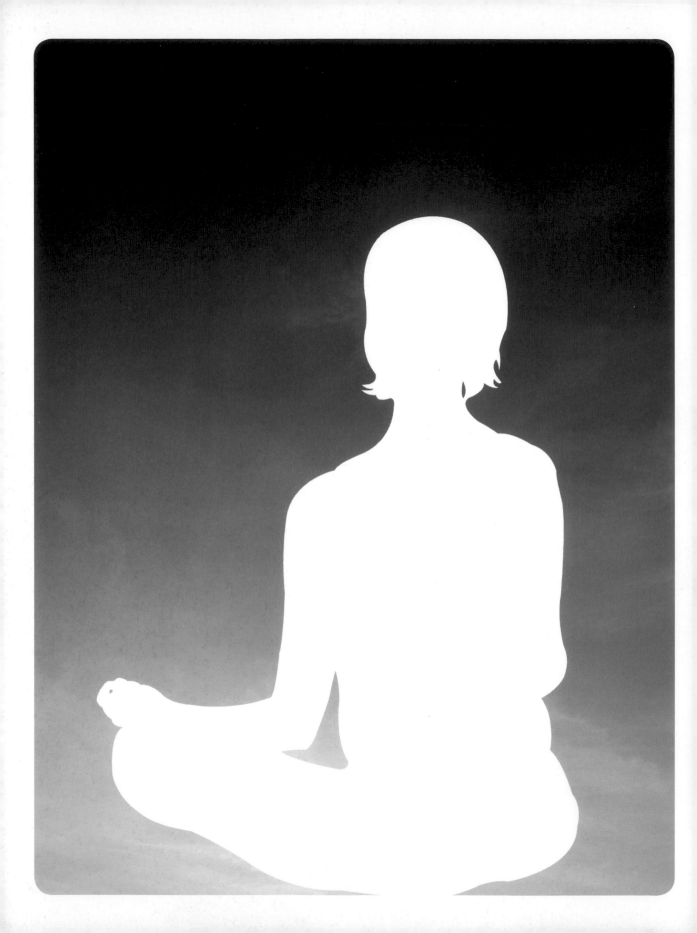

Basic practices

The first steps on any journey are often the most important. To get the most out of your yoga practice, you first need to learn how to breathe and relax properly. The importance of this cannot be over emphasized. Breathing and relaxing correctly lays a strong foundation on which to then build your practice. For the yoga postures to have maximum benefit, breathing needs to be conscious and married hand in hand with movement. Take your time and enjoy learning.

Getting started

To get the most out of yoga, you first need to learn how to breathe and relax properly. The yogic science of controlling the breath is known as *pranayama* and its main aim is the control of *prana* – the energy that lies behind each and every action. We can go without food and water for some time, but breath is the food that keeps the spark of life in us. As such, the movement of this energy through breathing is central to all yoga practices and there are yogic breathing exercises designed to teach control of the breath (see pages 24–7).

The state of your breathing reflects your state of mind. It also has a direct effect on the nervous system. Just as yoga poses directly tone the physical body, *pranayama* breathing exercises tone and strengthens the nervous system. By balancing the breath, thoughts are regulated, the emotions are balanced, we are relaxed, stress free and full of energy.

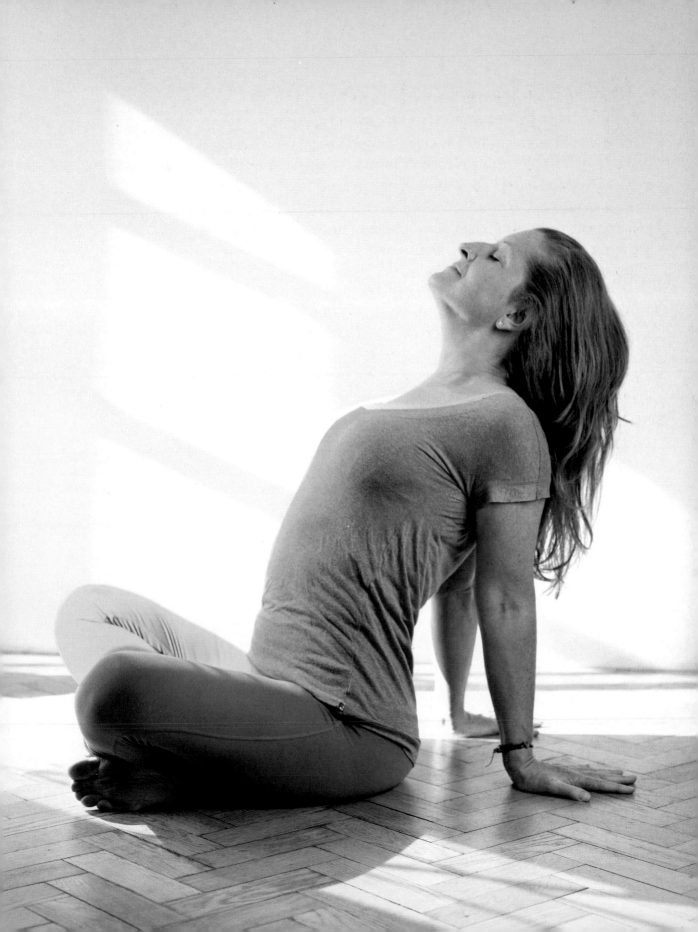

Breathing correctly

The main muscle associated with the action of breathing is the diaphragm. It is a dome-shaped muscle that separates the chest from the abdomen and is connected at the sternum and at the bottom of the ribcage. On inhalation, the diaphragm is pulled downward and flattened. At the same time, the muscles of the rib cage contract, the chest expands and lifts and air is drawn into the lungs to fill the expanded space in the chest cavity. On exhalation, the diaphragm relaxes and is pushed up, becoming dome-shaped again. The ribcage lowers as the muscles between the ribs relax. This decreased volume in the chest causes the air to be pushed out of the lungs.

guru guide

• Make the inhalation and exhalation of equal length.

• Work with your eyes closed and relax your body.

Practise this slow steady breathing for 2–3 minutes.

Abdominal breathing

Learning how to breathe deeply and fully is the first step and key to your yoga practice. Make your breath slow and full and focus on the movement of your abdomen.

Be aware of the movement in your rib cage, your lower back and kidney region, and the sensations in the back of your body against the ground. Notice how you feel when you practise.

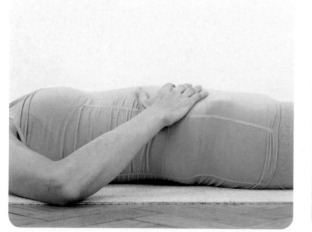

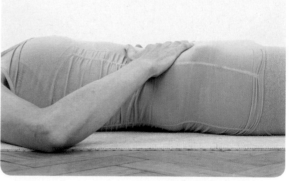

1 Lie on your back with your feet about 60 cm (2 ft) apart. Place your hands on your abdomen and allow your elbows to rest to the side. As you inhale through your nose, notice the rising of your abdomen, how your hands are lifted and fingers separate. Count to 4 as you inhale, making your breathing slow and rhythmical.

2 On the exhalation notice how the abdomen draws back and your hands move down, fingers coming closer together. Exhale for a count of 4. Practise this slow steady breathing for 2–3 minutes.

Full yogic breath

Once you feel comfortable with abdominal breathing, move on to practise full yogic breath. Making full use of the respiratory system in a controlled conscious way feeds your muscles with oxygen as you move in and out of postures, making them more efficient, stronger and flexible. It also reduces the build-up of lactic acid and stiffness in the body associated with physical exercise. Furthermore, full yogic breath has a deeply relaxing effect on the mind as it connects you to your body, developing and fine-tuning your bodily awareness.

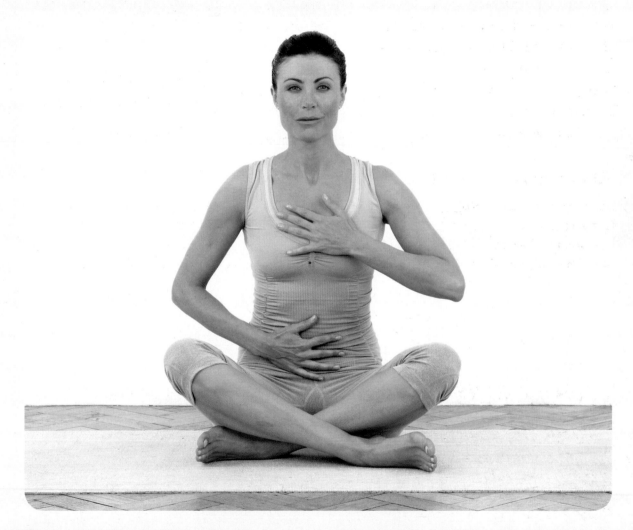

1 In a comfortable crossed-leg seated position (see page 33), place one hand on your abdomen and the other hand on your chest. Inhale deeply through your nose and notice the expansion in your abdomen, then your rib cage, your chest and, finally, how your top hand rises. Exhale and allow first the abdomen to relax, then your rib cage and, last, your chest. Gently contract your abdomen to empty your lungs completely of air. Practise breathing like this for 2–3 minutes and then release your hands and continue for a further minute with your eyes closed, focusing on your breath and the movement of your abdomen, ribcage and chest.

Alternate nostril breathing

Alternate nostril breathing (*anuloma viloma*) is energizing and brings a state of mental concentration, focus and calm. *Anuloma* means 'regular', and *viloma* means 'interrupted'. The left nostril is the path of cooling energy, and the right nostril that of heating energy, so through this practice the natural breath is balanced, therefore balancing the energy in your body.

Start with 3–5 rounds of alternate nostril breathing and build to 20 rounds over time. As you develop your practice, incorporate breathing with retention and gradually increase the count ratio to 5:10 and then 6:12. Begin with 5–6 rounds and build up to 10 rounds. You can then increase the count ratio to 5:10:20 and then 6:24:12.

guru guide

• Work at a pace you feel comfortable with.

• *Vishnu mudra* is formed by folding the index and middle fingers and keeping the thumb, ring and little fingers straight.

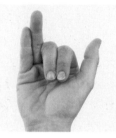

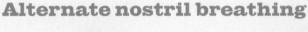

Alternate nostril breathing

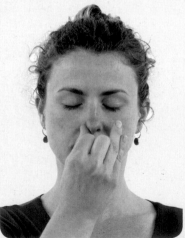

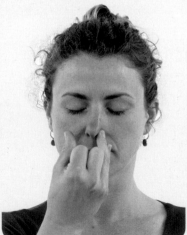

1 Sitting, preferably cross-legged, rest your left hand on the back of your left knee in *chin mudra* (see page 151) and your right hand in *vishnu mudra* (see above). Close your eyes and breathe deeply. Close your right nostril with your right thumb and inhale for a count of 4 through the left nostril.

2 Remove your thumb, place your ring finger over the left nostril and exhale for a count of 8 through the right nostril. Inhale through the right for 4, remove your ring finger and replace your thumb on your right nostril and then exhale through the left for a count of 8. This is 1 round.

With retention

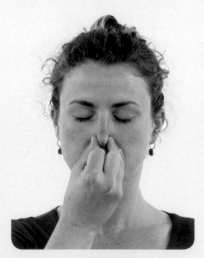

1 Breathe as for alternate nostril breathing, but between inhaling and exhaling, close both nostrils and retain your breath for a count of 16. If the retention is too much, start with a count of 8.

Shining skull breath KAPALABHATI

Once you have mastered alternate nostril breathing with breath retention, you can start to practise shining skull breath. As well as all the benefits of more basic breathing, the pumping action of this *pranayama* tones your abdominal muscles and gives a gentle massage to your internal organs. The forced exhalation also rids the lungs of stale air and makes space for fresh oxygen-rich breath.

As you feel comfortable with *kapalabhati* gradually increase the number of pumps to 60 per round. Increase the speed of the breath up to one pump per second. As your capacity increases, extend the length of the retentions, working up to 60–90 seconds. Focus your internal gaze between your eyebrows, the third eye, which is sometimes referred to as the seat of intuition.

guru guide

• Keep your chest and shoulders relaxed; the movement comes from the abdomen.

• If you feel dizzy, stop and lie down. Make sure you are not pumping too fast.

• Focus on the heat that is being created in your abdomen, stimulating the movement of energy in your body.

Start by practising
3 rounds of
20 pumps.

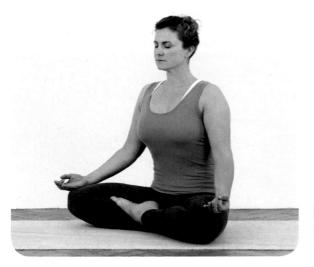

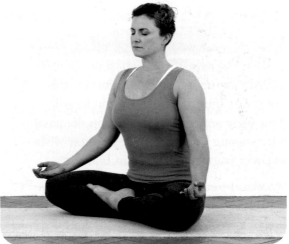

1 Sit in a comfortable seated position (see page 33 or sit on a chair with your feet flat on the ground, back straight and away from the chair back). Rest your hands on the backs on your knees in *chin mudra* (see page 151). Take a couple of deep breaths to prepare. Inhale and then exhale forcefully through both nostrils, simultaneously drawing back your abdomen.

2 Relax your abdomen and allow the inhalation to occur naturally. Repeat the exhalation and inhalation 20 times, finishing on an active exhale. Then take two slow full yogic breaths, before inhaling to three-quarters lung capacity and retaining the breath. Hold for as long as you can without strain and slowly exhale. Take two full yogic breaths before beginning the next round. Start by practising 3 rounds of 20 pumps.

Relaxation poses

Relaxation poses are used before, during and at the end of practice. They relax the nervous and respiratory systems and re-energize the body and mind.

Child's pose BALASANA

Child's pose relaxes the spine and stretches out the lower back. It quietens the mind as the centre of the forehead gently touches the earth. Child's pose is the counter pose to headstand and back bending poses. It can also be done when a pause is needed during your practice, as it rejuvenates and energizes the whole body.

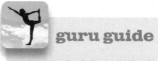

guru guide

• Let your body be completely still and relaxed. Focus on your breathing and be aware of its natural rhythm.

Breathe deeply and **rhythmically** for at least **5 breaths.**

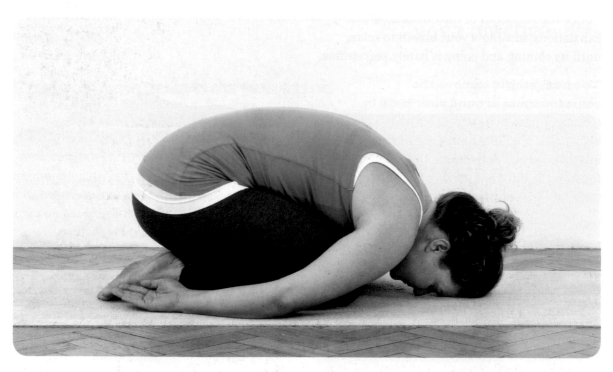

1 Kneel down and fold your body forward, placing your forehead on the ground. Relax your shoulders and place the backs of your hands alongside your feet. Breathe deeply and rhythmically for at least 5 breaths. In particular, hold child's pose for at least 5 breaths after headstand (see pages 116–17) and for 1–2 minutes after any back bends (see pages 82–93 and 126–35).

Corpse pose SAVASANA

Corpse pose is often deemed the hardest *asana* to perform because you lie as still as a 'corpse' and relax as you remain conscious and aware; this develops awareness of the mind and deepens the process of relaxation as described on pages 28–9.

This pose has a profound effect on the whole body mind system. Use it at the beginning and end of your practice and you can also use it can during a session, particularly after dynamic practices as it calms the breath and energizes the body, relaxing the nerves and removing fatigue.

guru guide

- Let your body be completely still and relaxed, while focusing on your breathing.

Focus on your breathing for at least 2 minutes.

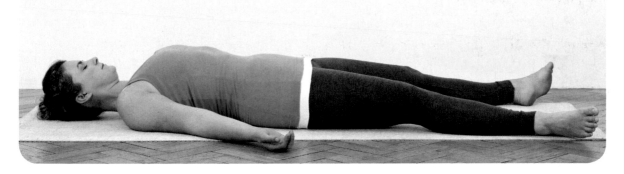

1 Lie flat on your back with your feet about 60 cm (2 ft) apart, arms away from the sides of your body and your palms facing up and relaxed, allowing your fingers to gently curl. Imagine a line between the crown of your head and your heels and visualize the symmetry of your body. Slide your shoulders down the back of your body and relax your neck. Move your focus towards your breath. Become aware of your natural breath, its rhythm, depth and sensations accompanying inhalation and exhalation. Focus on your breathing for at least 2 minutes.

For comfort

If your back feels uncomfortable lying flat on the ground, as shown above, practise corpse pose with your knees bent and feet hip-width apart on the floor. This position will be more comfortable for your lower back as it relaxes into the ground.

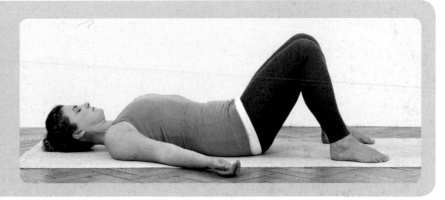

Preparation for practice

Yoga is about practice. It demands time and commitment and you have to do it to understand it. It doesn't matter at what point in your life you start, young or old, but once you have made the decision to begin, then begin. Yoga makes you stronger, more flexible and improves your breathing, but the real gems lie inside and what you get from yoga is so much more than you could ever imagine.

guru guide

• It can be helpful to keep a diary of your practice, making notes of what you have done and how you felt. Over time you will be able to see your progression and the areas that you could spend more time on.

Setting your intention

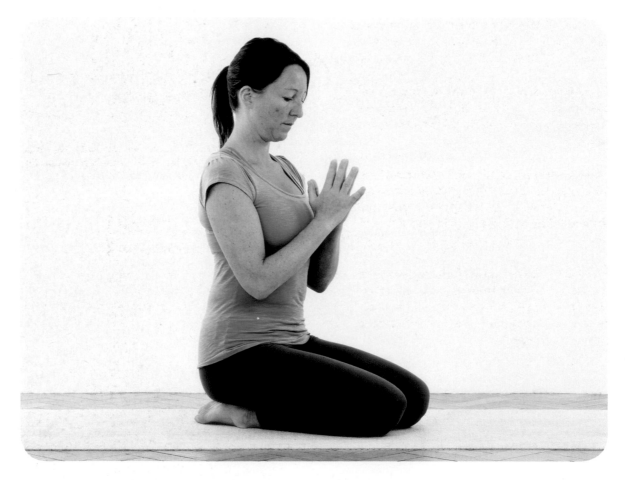

One of the key principles of yoga is a dedication of your actions. Dedicate your practice to someone or something that is of inspiration to you. In this way you elevate your practice as a service to a cause greater than yourself.

Making the most of your time

When preparing for and doing yoga, there are a few things that are important to consider:

You can practise at any time of the day, but do it on an empty stomach, waiting 2–3 hours after a heavy meal.

If you can find a regular time that works for you, this is particularly advantageous.

Choose a time and place where you can practise undisturbed by phone calls or other duties.

Wear clothes that are comfortable and easy to move in – natural fabrics that allow your body to breath are best.

Practise on a yoga mat and have a cushion and blanket to hand for sitting and relaxation. It is important to be comfortable and not push, or strain.

The postures are about finding balance; they create symmetry in your body and create a balanced state of mind. Make sure that your practice is balanced so if you do something on the right side, ensure you also do it on the left.

The key to success is little and often, it is better to do a small amount on a regular basis than practising for hours once in a blue moon – but something is always better than nothing, so roll out your mat and begin.

Practise little and often and somewhere you can be comfortable and remain uninterrupted.

Making yourself comfortable

Many of the practices in the beginner chapter (see pages 34–59) can be done from a sitting or kneeling position.

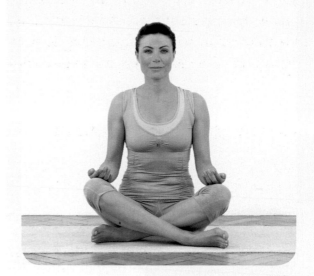

Sitting cross-legged: Sit on the floor and cross your legs at the shins. Have your spine, neck and head in line. Sit on a cushion if it is helpful.

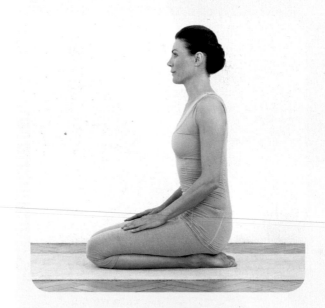

Kneeling: If there is too much pressure on your knees, place a cushion between your heels and your buttocks.

Leg exercises STRETCHING AND RAISING

◆ GOOD FOR: Flexibility in your legs and hips

These stretches are particularly focused on leg and hip flexibility and abdominal and lower back strength as they stretch the hips and hamstring muscles. They also encourage the flow of energy in the body and develop rhythmical and deep breathing while holding a stretch.

guru guide

• Keep your lower back pressed down and into the floor and your leg straight.

• Remember to take full deep breaths throughout.

Head to knee stretch

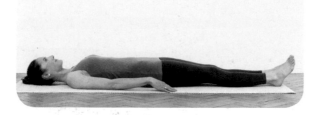

1 Lie flat on you your back with your legs straight and together. Place your arms by your sides, palms facing down and with your head straight and chin very gently drawn in towards the chest.

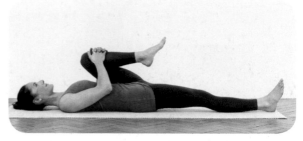

2 Bend your left knee and draw it close to your chest. Clasp your hands over the top of the shin. Gently press the back of your right leg towards the floor. Exhale as you draw your left knee close to your chest.

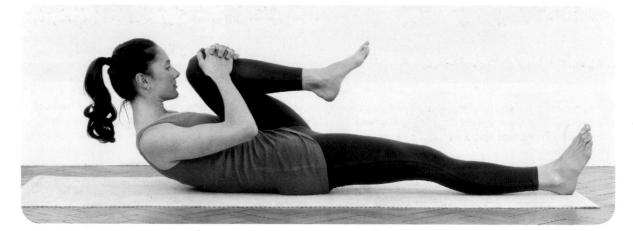

3 Inhale and lift up your head and chest, touching your nose as close to your left knee as you can. Hold for a couple of breaths and then slowly exhale and lower your head and chest back down. Place your hands by your sides and lower your left leg down onto the mat. Do the same with the right leg. Repeat 3 times.

Hip stretch

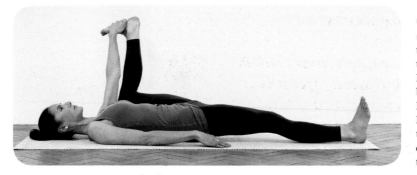

1 Start as step 1, opposite. Draw your left knee into your chest, then slide the top of your thigh towards the left side of your body. Raise your foot up, keeping your knee bent and, with your left hand, take hold of the inside edge of your foot. Focus on drawing the top of your left thigh towards the ground on the exhalations. Hold for 6 breaths and then repeat with your right leg.

Single leg raises

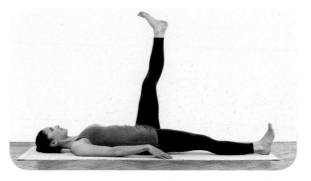

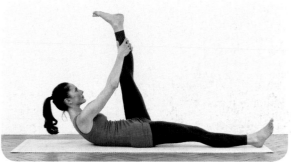

1 Lie as for the head to knee stretch. Inhale and raise your left leg, lifting it as far as you can towards 90 degrees and keeping both legs straight. Exhale and lower your left leg. Inhale and raise your right leg, exhale and lower it. Do this 6 times for each leg.

2 Inhale and raise your left leg, then, as you exhale, take hold of your leg and lift your head and chest off the floor, raising your chest up towards the lifted leg. Keep both of your legs straight and focus on deep rhythmical breaths. Hold for 6 breaths and repeat with the right leg.

Double leg raises

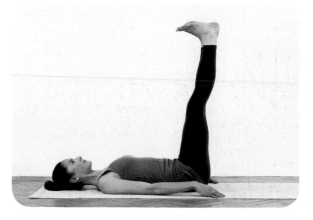

Repeat each exercise as instructed.

1 Lie as for the head to knee stretch. Inhale and raise both legs up to 90 degrees, keeping them straight and together. Keep your lower back down on the ground. Exhale and lower your legs. Repeat up to 10 times and then relax in the corpse pose (see page 31) for a few breaths.

Bridge SETU BANDASANA

◆ GOOD FOR: Releasing tension in your back, neck and shoulders

Setu is a 'bridge' and *bandha* means 'formation', so this pose means that it resembles the construction of a bridge. The pose realigns the spine and makes it supple, while opening the chest. It also prepares the body for the more challenging back bends on pages 82–93 and 126–35.

Repeat up to 5 times.

guru guide

• You can also work dynamically in bridge pose, inhaling the hips up and exhaling them down, working with breath and movement. You could do this for 6 inhales and 6 exhalations.

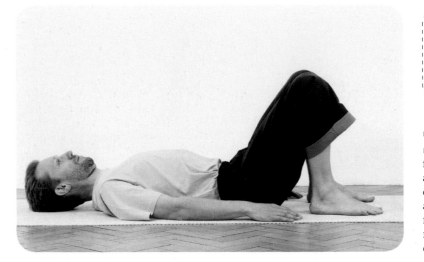

> *Related pose*
>
> Shoulderstand to bridge (pages 122–3)

1 Lie flat on your back and bend your knees, placing your feet flat on the floor so they are parallel and hip-width apart. Place your heels directly under your knees. Have your arms alongside your body, palms facing down, and the back of your neck long and your chin gently drawn in towards your chest.

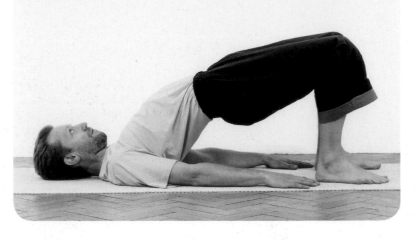

2 Inhale and lift up your hips, keeping your knees hip-width apart and outside edges of the thighs gently rolling in. Press your hands and arms gently down and lift your upper chest up and back towards your chin. Feel the arch and lift through the back of your body. Hold for as long as you can and then on an exhalation lower your body. Repeat up to 5 times.

Lying twist JATHARA PARIVRTANASANA

◆ GOOD FOR: Releasing tension from your back and spine

Jathara is translated as 'stomach', 'abdomen' or 'bowels' and *parivrtana* means 'turning around' or 'rolling'. This simple supine twist is a wonderful pose for stimulating digestion and relieving digestive tract complaints as it massages the abdominal organs. It is also a precursor to the twists on pages 96–9 and 136–7.

guru guide

• Keep the backs of your shoulders down, chest open and length in the side of your body.

• This pose can also be practised as a dynamic movement with breath. Take one breath to one movement, exhaling the knees to the sides and inhaling to the centre. When practising in this way, repeat 3 times on each side.

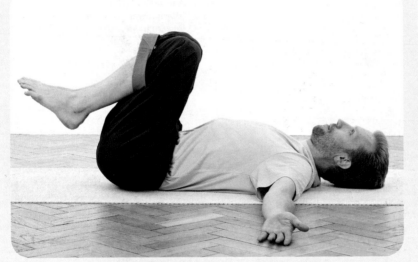

1 Lie on your back and extend your arms wide at shoulder height. Inhale and bend your knees into your chest. Keep your head straight and in line with your spine; chin in towards your chest.

Hold the pose for up to 1 minute on each side.

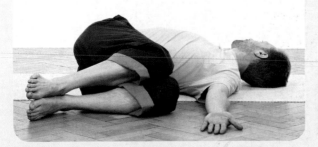

2 Exhale as you bring your knees to the left and turn your head to the right. Hold the pose and then inhale, bringing your knees and then your head back to the centre.

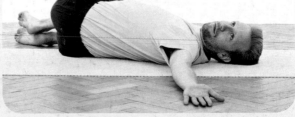

3 Exhale and take your knees over to the right and turn your head to the left. Hold the pose for up to 1 minute on each side.

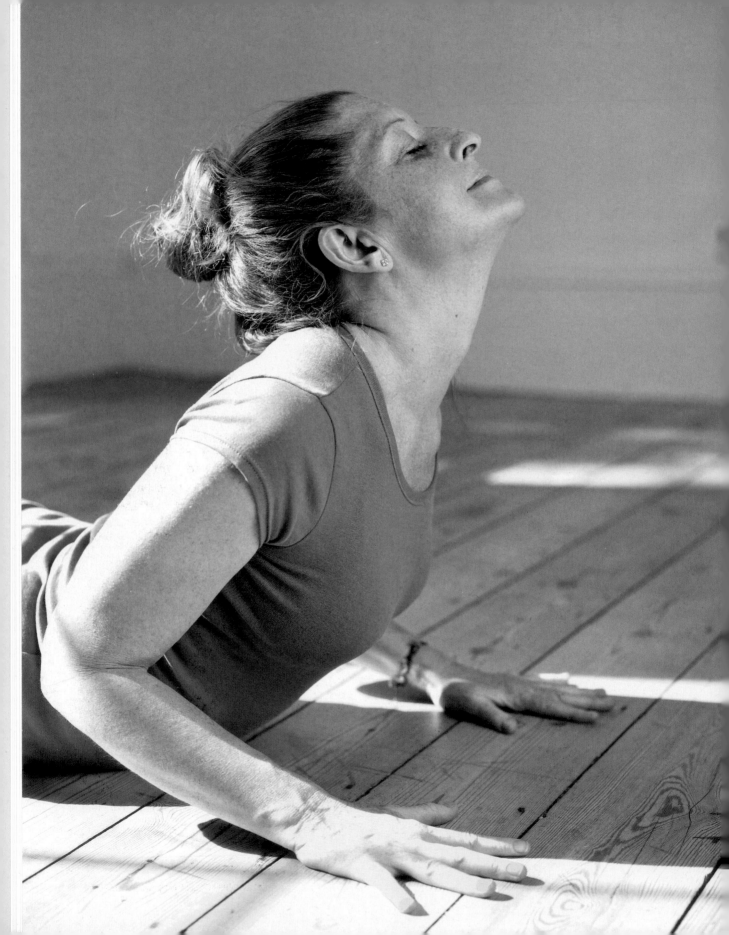

Introducing the sun salutation SURYA NAMASKAR

The sun salutation is a series of 12 physical movements comprising alternating backward and forward bending poses that bring flexion and extension to the spinal column and limbs.

As such, it is a complete practice. It can be seen as a prayer to the sun and our own inner light: *surya* translates as 'sun' and *namaskar* as 'salutation'. The 12 movements also represent the 12 months of the year as well as the 12 signs of the zodiac. It is the ideal way to start your practice, especially in the morning at sunrise.

A prayer to the sun

From the dawning of time, the sun has been a symbol of worship. Practises directed to the energy of the sun have been around for thousands of years, to honour and acknowledge its life-giving force and grace. The sun is a symbol for many things health and life giving.

Surya was the name given to the sun god of ancient India, and the practice of *surya namaskar* is referred to in early scriptures and recommended as part of daily spiritual practice. The Greeks built temples in the sun's honour, worshipping the Sun God, Apollo. The practise of *surya namaskar* therefore connects us to ancient traditions of reverence for the sun and to our dependence on the fiery ball that daily rises in the sky.

Surya namaskar is one of the most integrated yogic practices. It has the benefit of both *asanas* and *pranayama* and the attitude with which it is performed can bring tremendous concentration, developing the practice into a moving meditation. Sun salutation also presents many advantages for the different aspects of ourselves.

Physically it removes stiffness from the body, increases flexibility and exercises the leg and arm muscles.

Deep breathing is encouraged and mental sluggishness removed. It fosters peace of mind by concentrating on the rhythmical systematic movement of the body and breath.

Practised with an attitude of devotion and prayer it purifies the heart and mind. Traditionally practised with mantras for celebrating aspects of the sun's divinity, it is the mental attitude, focus and concentration that are most important.

Sun salutation surya namaskar

◆ GOOD FOR: Flexibility of your spine

As explained on page 63, the sun salutation is a dynamic series of 12 movements flowing into each other, which combine to exercise the whole body. It is described over these two pages and overleaf.

Familiarize yourself with each step and then start by practising steps 1, 2, 3, 10, 11 and 12. Then work with the transition between steps 3 and 4 and 8 and 9. You can then work with steps 4, 5, 6, 7, 8, and 9 together. Once you have mastered the two sequences, it makes the whole series of movements flow more easily.

Start by practising 2–3 rounds of the sun salutation and build it up to 12 rounds as you develop confidence and your physical ability improves.

Preparation

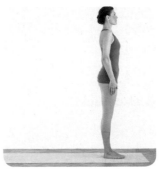

• Stand at the front of the mat with your feet together and arms by your sides. Be aware of your feet on the floor, weight equally distributed. Feel the crown of your head lifting up, elongating your spine.

The sun salutation

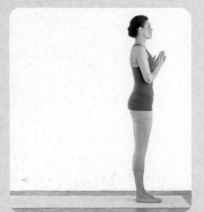

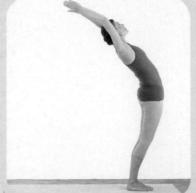

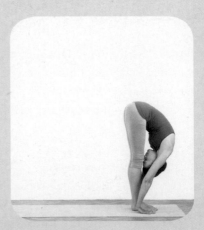

1 Stand erect, feet together. Bring your palms together in the centre of your chest. Exhale fully and be aware of the sensation created between your palms. Keep your breast bone lifted.

2 Inhale and stretch both hands up and over your head. Face your palms forward and have your arms shoulder-width apart. Push your hips forward and arch back. Feel the stretch in your upper back.

3 Exhale and bend forward from your hips until your hands are on the mat with your fingers in line with your toes. If necessary, bend your knees to get your hands on the floor. Draw your chest towards your thighs.

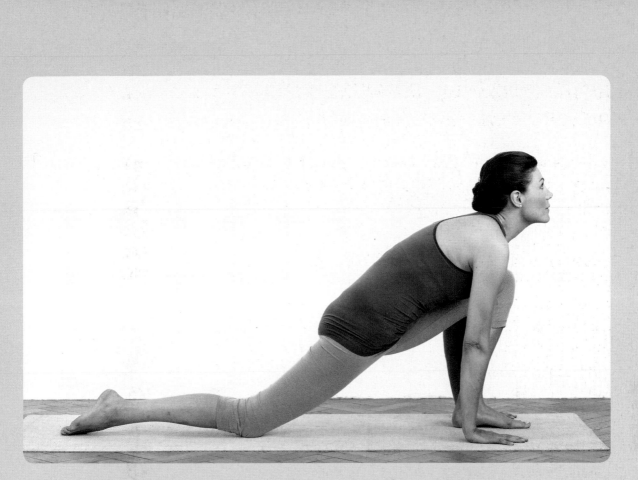

4 Keeping your hands on the floor, inhale and step your right leg all the way back so that your right knee and foot are on the floor. Let your pelvis come forward, arch your spine and look up. Focus on the stretch in your thigh.

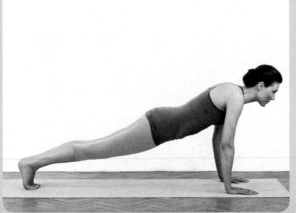

5 Hold your breath as you tuck your toes on the right foot under, straighten your right leg and take your left leg back, into plank. Keep your back straight and your neck in line. Direct your gaze towards the floor.

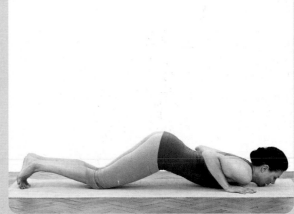

6 Exhaling, lower your knees, then chest and chin or forehead onto the floor. Keep your hips up and elbows in so your knees, hands, chest and chin touch the floor and your spine is arched. (Turn to pages 66–7 for steps 7–12.)

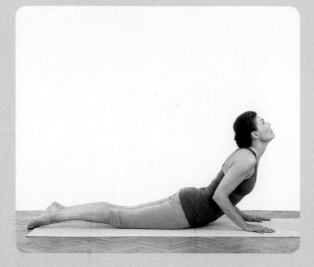

7 On the inhalation, stretch and arch your body forward and up so that your hips and legs stay on the ground. Keep your shoulders away from your ears and elbows in. Look up.

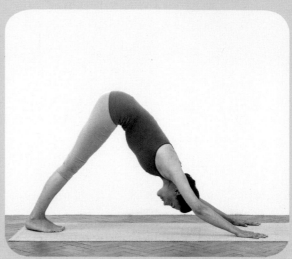

8 Tuck your toes under and, exhaling, lift your hips and push your heels down towards the floor, drawing your chest back towards your thighs. Keep your head relaxed. The body should form a triangle with the ground in this inverted 'V' pose.

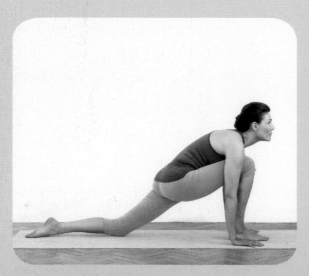

9 Inhaling, bring your right foot forward between your hands and put your left knee down on the floor. Push your pelvis forward, lift your chest and look up.

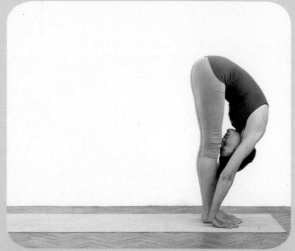

10 Exhaling, bring your left leg forward next to the right. With your fingertips and toes in line, try to straighten your legs, as in step 3. Draw your chest towards your thighs.

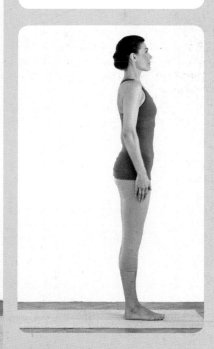

guru guide

• Avoid strain and relax in each position.

• Let the movements flow, flexing forward and back, bringing maximum benefit to your spinal column.

• The benefits of sun salutation are many. It:
Regulates breathing
Increases flexibility in your
    spine and limbs
Develops mental focus and
    concentration
Helps overcome stiffness in the
    body and joints
Develops sensitivity to the body
Fosters a sense of joy and
    wellbeing.

11 Inhale and stretch forward and up and then arch your body back with the palms of your hands facing each other.

12 Exhale and bring your arms by your sides. Take a deep inhalation and then exhale as you start again with step 1. This time take the left leg back in step 4 and your right knee to the ground in step 9.

Shoulderstand SARVANGASANA

◆ GOOD FOR: Strengthening your spine

The shoulderstand is an inverted pose that nourishes the whole body (*sarva* means 'whole' and *anga* means 'body') as it stimulates and balances the thyroid glands, promoting a balancing effect. It also draws fresh oxygenated blood down into the skull and brain. It is sometimes known as the queen or mother of the *asanas*.

> *Related poses*
>
> Plough (pages 70–1)
>
> Fish (pages 72–3)
>
> Shoulderstand to bridge (pages 122–3)

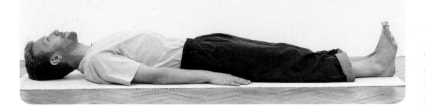

1 Lie on your back, legs together and arms by the sides of your body, palms facing down into the floor. Your neck should be long, so have your chin slightly drawn in towards your chest.

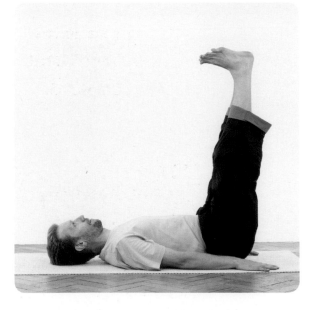

2 On an inhalation raise your legs, keeping your feet flexed and your back pressed into the floor.

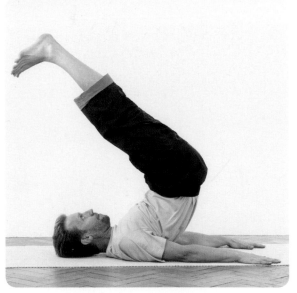

3 Continue to inhale as you lift up your hips and chest. Your arms can support this movement by gently pressing down into the floor.

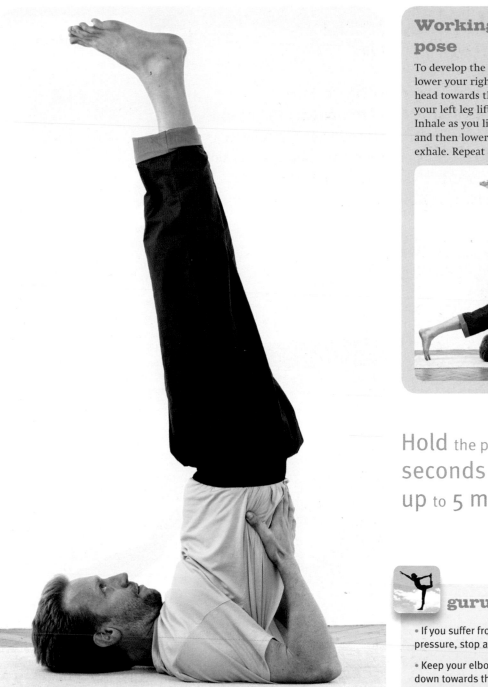

To develop the pose, exhale and lower your right leg behind your head towards the floor. Keep your left leg lifted straight up. Inhale as you lift the leg back up and then lower the left leg on an exhale. Repeat a few times.

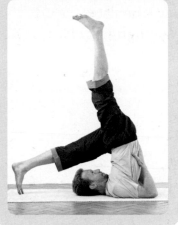

Hold the pose for 45 seconds and build up to 5 minutes.

guru guide

• If you suffer from high blood pressure, stop at step 2.

• Keep your elbows in and hands down towards the upper back, this makes it easy to balance and brings your body straighter.

• Keep your head relaxed and straight and your legs and feet together.

4 Support your back with your hands, your elbows in line with your shoulders and hands on your back, fingers pointing up to your waist. Draw your chest back towards your chin and align your hips above your shoulders. Once you are steady, hold the pose for 45 seconds and build up to 5 minutes.

intermediate practices 69

Seated forward bend PASCHIMOTANASANA

◆ GOOD FOR: Stretching your hamstrings and flexing your hip joints

A forward bend, *paschima* means the 'west', or back of the body, so this is a pose that stretches the back of the body. As circulation is increased in the spine, the spinal nerves are flooded with oxygen, releasing physical and mental tension. A deep massage is placed on the internal organs and the kidney region is stretched, toning the abdominal region and removing excess weight. It is beneficial for menstrual complaints and sluggish digestion and also has a meditative quality, as it teaches us to surrender to the power of breath in a challenging situation.

After completing this pose or a series of seated forward bends (see pages 76–9), practise the incline plane (see page 80) as a counter pose.

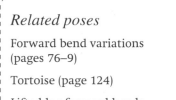

Related poses

Forward bend variations
(pages 76–9)

Tortoise (page 124)

Lifted leg forward bends
(page 125)

At first, hold the pose for 5–6 breaths and gradually work up to 5 minutes.

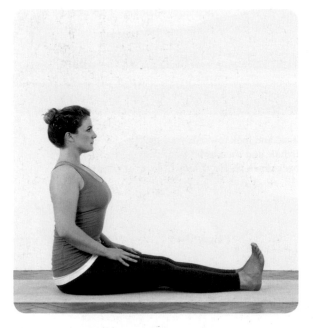

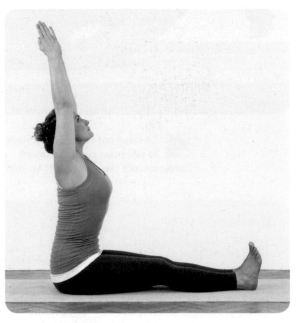

1 Sit with your legs stretched out in front of you, legs and feet together and your spine straight. Gently flex your feet so the toes point back towards you.

2 Inhale and stretch your arms straight up above your head, keeping them in line with your ears. Lift up your body from the hips and feel the side of your waist lengthen. Lift your gaze slightly up.

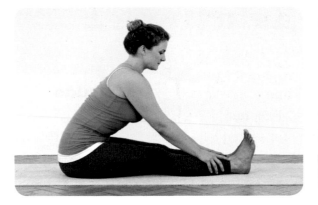

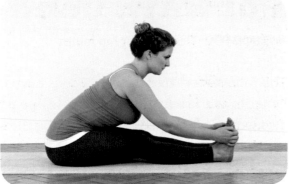

3 Exhale and bend forward from your hips. Reach with your hands as far as you can and hold your ankles or calves. Keep your spine and head in alignment. Hold for 5–6 breaths and repeat up to 3 times, gradually increasing the time spent in the pose. As you gain more flexibility you can move onto step 4. Come out of the pose on an inhalation.

4 Starting from step 2, exhale and fold forward from your hips. Take hold of your feet, and draw your chest down towards your legs. Use your breath to work in the pose and as you hold and focus on long exhalations relax into the stretch and work on bringing your head and chest closer to your legs.

guru guide

• Stretch forward from your hips for maximum benefit.

• COMMON MISTAKES TO AVOID (see below): don't round your upper back, bend your head to your chest, or have your legs apart and feet inactive.

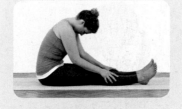

5 To come into the full pose, exhale and fold forward and then take hold of your big toes with your index fingers. Take your elbows towards the floor and forehead to your shins, bringing your abdomen to rest completely on your thighs. For maximum benefit, work up to holding this pose for 5 minutes.

Working in the pose

Once you are comfortable with the full pose you can try variations. Stretch your arms forward and bring your palms together. Flex your toes towards your knees and rest your arms on the toes. Remain active in the pose to get a deep stretch.

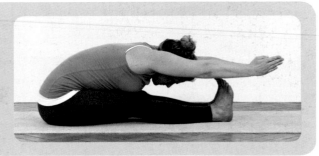

Forward bend variations 2

◆ GOOD FOR: Flexibility in your hamstrings, hips and spine

These seated forward bends have a relaxing effect on the mind and release the build-up of tension in the back from prolonged sitting or standing. To get more out of the forward bends, place emphasis on exhalation, which is associated with our ability to let go, releasing mental and physical stiffness. The side bend with twist also stretches the waist and opens the thoracic spine. You have to rotate the chest at the same time as bending to the side, freeing the lower back and opening the hips. Both the exercises also relax the nervous system very effectively.

Related poses

Seated forward bends
(pages 74–7)

Tortoise (page 124)

Lifted leg forward bends
(page 125)

Hold each part of the pose as instructed.

Forward bend with legs wide

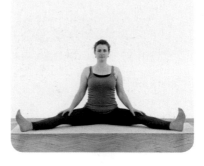

1 Sit with your legs stretched as wide apart as you can. Keep your feet active and toes pointing up.

guru guide

• These exercises are a good preparation for the body to sit for meditation.

• In the side bend with twist, rotate your chest upwards.

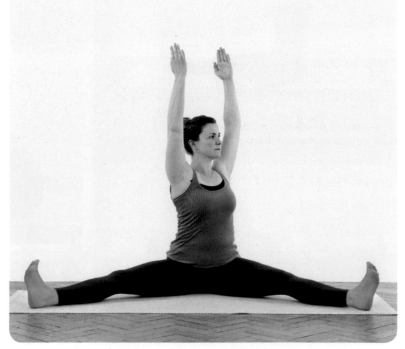

2 Inhale and stretch your arms up above your head, palms facing each other and turning your body towards the left side. Lift up and out of your hips and reach tall though your arms.

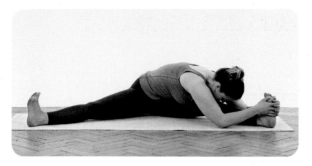

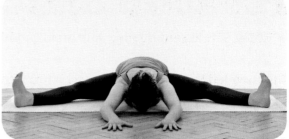

3 Exhale and bend forward, bringing your chest over your left leg. Take hold of your left foot and keep your head and neck relaxed. Hold for 1–2 minutes and then repeat on the other side.

4 Sitting as in step 1, inhale and stretch your arms up. Exhale and bend from your hips. Place your hands on the floor and bring your chest towards the ground. Focus on extending forward from your hips. Hold for 1 minute, then inhale and come back up, or continue to step 5.

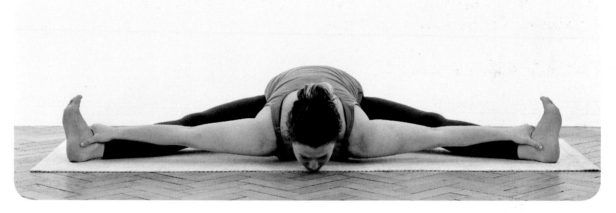

5 Reaching your arms wide, hold your ankles and, with each exhalation, bring your chest closer to the floor. Keep your legs and feet active. Hold the position for 1 minute, then inhale to release and come out of the pose.

Side bend with twist

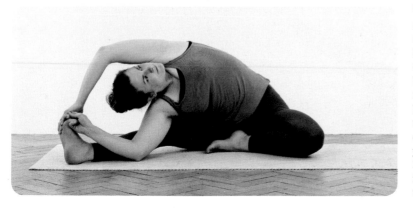

1 Sit as in step 1, opposite. Bend your left leg and bring the sole of the foot against your right thigh. Inhale and stretch both arms up, exhale as you twist and bend your body to the right. Reach with your right hand and take hold of the right big toe with your index finger and thumb. Bring your right elbow as close as you can to the floor. Stretch your left arm over your head and take hold of the outside edge of your right foot. Hold for 1–2 minutes. Repeat on the other side.

Incline plane PURVOTTANASANA

◆ GOOD FOR: Strengthening your arms and wrists

Incline plane should be done as a counter pose following any forward bends. *Purva* is the 'east', or the front of the body, so after the forward bends stretching the *paschima* (or back part of the body), the incline plane balances their effect and opens out the front side of the body west. If lifting your hips with your legs straight is too much, start with table top, opposite.

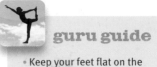

guru guide

• Keep your feet flat on the ground and relax your neck to stretch the front of the throat.

• Keep your breathing rhythmical.

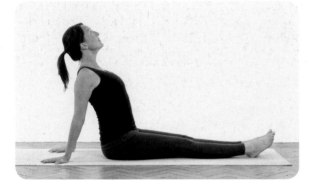

1 With your legs stretched in front of you and together, place your hands on the ground behind you, fingers pointing to the back of the mat and about shoulder-width apart and 30 cm (12 in) away from your body. Press into your hands as you expand your chest forward.

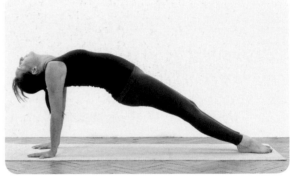

2 Inhale and lift your hips, chest out and take your head back, relaxing the neck. Press your feet flat into the ground and keep your legs straight. Hold for 8 breaths and then exhale as you lower the body down. Once you feel steady and confident in the pose try the arm and leg raises.

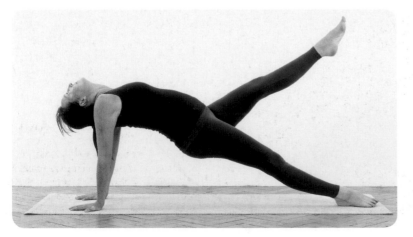

Hold each part of the pose as instructed.

3 From step 2, inhale and lift up your leg. Exhale it down and then repeat on the other leg. Do up to 3 times on each side.

Making it easier: table top

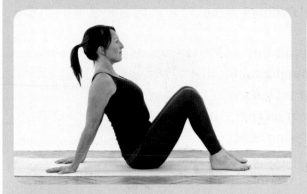

1 Sit with your legs in front of you and place your hands on the ground behind you, fingers pointing to the back of the mat and about shoulder-width apart and 30 cm (12 in) away from your body. Bend your knees and have your feet flat on the floor and hip-width apart.

2 Inhale and lift your hips, raising your thighs parallel to the ground. Take your head back and relax your neck. Keep your feet flat and hips up. Hold and breathe deeply for up to 8 breaths, exhaling as you lower your body.

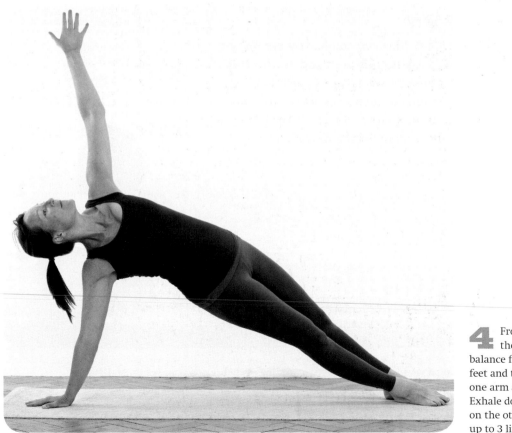

4 From step 2, press the weight and balance firmly into your feet and then inhale, raise one arm and look up. Exhale down and repeat on the other side doing up to 3 lifts on each arm.

Locust variations

◆ GOOD FOR: Strengthening your back and leg muscles

These poses give a deep diagonal stretch to the back of your body and massage the abdominal organs. They also stimulate your spinal nerves and develop coordination between movement and breath. Rest in crocodile (see page 82) between each variation and afterwards.

guru guide

• For the best stretch in these variations, lengthen your arms and legs and then lift them.

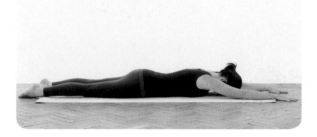

1 Lie flat on the on your stomach and stretch your arms forward and your legs back, together and straight. Rest your forehead on the floor.

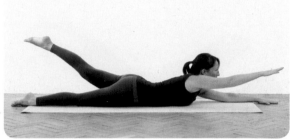

2 On an inhalation, lift your right arm and left leg, stretching your arms forward and leg back keeping them straight. Hold for a couple of breaths and then exhale and lower them. This is half a round. Repeat with the opposite arm and leg, completing up to 5 rounds.

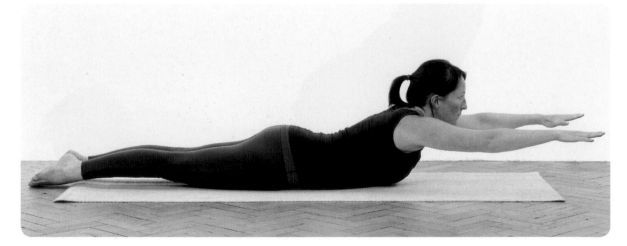

3 On an inhalation, lift up your arms, chest and head. Feel the front of your body stretching and lifting away from the floor. Keep your arms parallel to one another and your legs and feet together. Hold the pose for a couple of breaths and then, on an exhalation, lower the legs. Repeat 3 times.

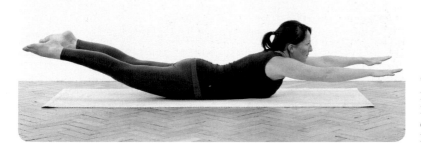

Related poses

Locust (pages 86–7)

Full locust (page 131)

4 Keep your arms straight in front of you, palms down and forehead on the floor. Inhale and lift your legs, extending the lower back and keeping your feet and legs together. Hold for a few breaths and then exhale and lower your legs. Repeat 3 times.

Repeat each
variation as
instructed.

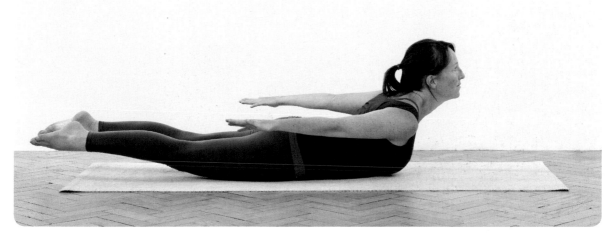

5 Inhaling, lift your arms, chest and head and, simultaneously, lift your legs, keeping them straight. Hold for as long as you can and then exhale and lower your legs and arms. Repeat 2–3 times.

6 Lie flat on your stomach and place your arms alongside your body, palms facing down and with your legs and feet together. Inhale and lift your head, chest, arms and legs as high as is comfortable. Hold the pose for as long as you can and exhale and come down. Repeat up to 3 times.

Bow DHANURASANA

◆ GOOD FOR: Strengthening your spine and expanding your chest

The bow is a back bend that makes the spine elastic like a bow. Strength and flexibility is also needed in the quadriceps to lift into and hold the bow. The abdominal organs and muscles are massaged, strengthening and soothing the digestive system and, at the same time, the mind is energized, encouraging mental alertness.

guru guide

• Try to lift your ribs and thighs away from the floor and keep your arms straight.

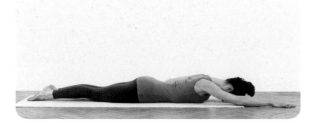

1 Lie on your front and stretch your right arm forward on the floor. Bend your left leg and reach back and take hold of the top of the foot with your left hand. Keep your forehead resting on the floor and ensure your neck is long and relaxed.

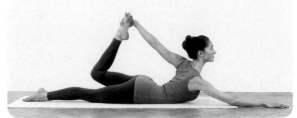

2 Inhale and simultaneously lift up your left leg and chest. Stretch your toes up and keep your left arm straight. Press your right hand and leg into the floor to ground the pose so you can lift the left side of your body higher. Hold for 5–6 breaths and repeat on the other side.

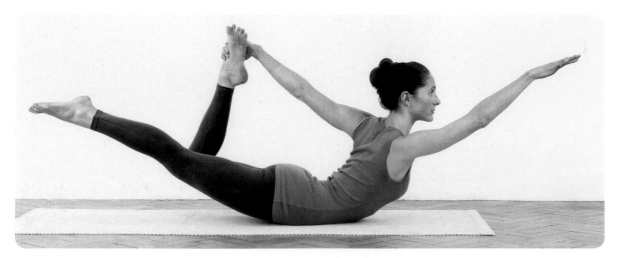

3 Position yourself again as in step 1. Inhaling, lift both arms and legs. Stretch your right arm forward and extend your right leg back. Hold your left foot, stretching the toes high. Lift your head and look forward. Balance your body around the navel. Hold for 5–6 breaths and exhale as you come down. Repeat on the other side.

Hold for 6 breaths and repeat up to 3 times.

Related pose
Full bow (page 135)

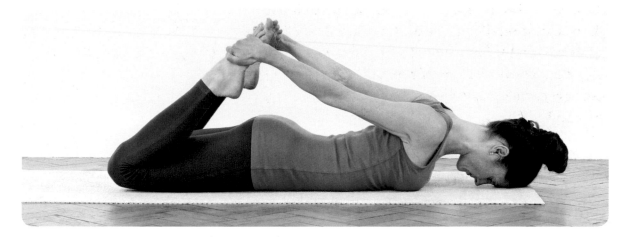

4 Again lying on your abdomen, as in step 1, bend both knees and reach back, taking hold of the tops of your feet (or your ankles if you find this easier). Keep your arms straight, your feet relaxed and rest your forehead on the floor.

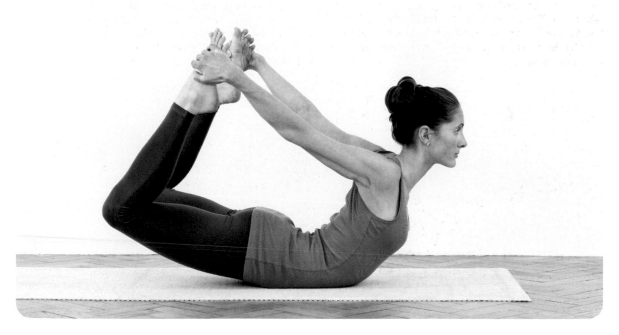

5 Inhale and lift your legs and chest, trying to get your thighs off the ground. Balance your body on your abdomen and, at the same time, lift up your head and look up, focusing on a point straight ahead of you. Hold for 6 breaths and repeat up to 3 times. Relax in crocodile (see page 82).

Crescent moon ANJANEYASANA

◆ GOOD FOR: Flexibility in your hips and spine

The full pose of this back bend resembles a semicircle
like the crescent moon and demands flexibility and
balance. Start by practising steps 1 and 2 and as you
build confidence work with step 3.

Related poses
Splits (pages 128–9)
Pigeon (pages 132–3)

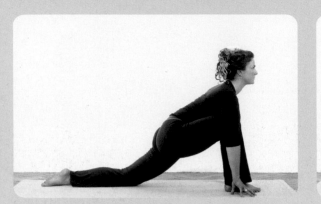

1 Come into a lunge position, bringing your right foot
forward between your hands and stretching your left
leg back. Sink your hips forward and lift your chest. Keep
your breath rhythmical.

2 Keeping your hips dropping close towards the floor,
inhale and bring your palms into prayer position.
Take 2 breaths and allow your hips to drop a little further
forward with your exhalations.

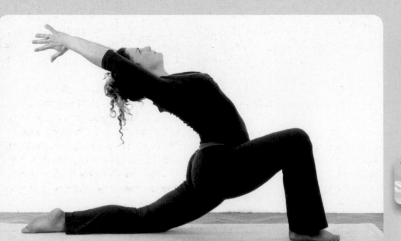

Hold the full crescent moon for 5 breaths.

guru guide

• Keep your pelvis forward and
down and feel the stretch in your
back thigh as you keep your arms
in alignment with your ears.

• Breathe deeply when holding
the pose and look up.

3 Inhale and lift your arms up above your head, gently arching your body.
Keep your arms straight and elbows drawing in. Exhale as you further arch
your body. Hold for 5 breaths and exhale as you release, bringing your hands
down onto the floor. Repeat on the other side. Relax in child's pose (see page 30).

Camel USTRASANA

◆ GOOD FOR: Mobilizing your neck, shoulders and back

Camel (a direct translation of the word *ustra*) is a great back bend for relieving a tight upper back and shoulders. It also stretches the thigh muscles and works on the digestive system stretching and massaging the stomach and intestines.

guru guide

• Keep your thighs perpendicular and at an angle of 90 degrees with the lower leg. Keep your pelvis forward and chest lifted.

• Relax your back muscles and focus on creating space in the thoracic spine.

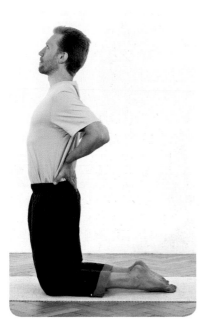

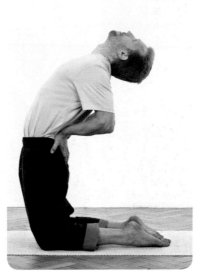

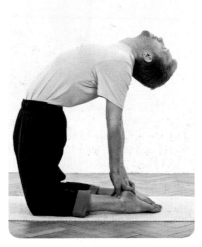

1 Kneel with your feet and knees hip-width apart. From the tip of your toes to the knees forms the base of the pose. Support your lower back with your hands, fingers facing down. Press your hips and tailbone slightly forward and keep your breath rhythmical.

2 Exhale and arch back, pressing the front of your thighs and hips forward. Feel the stretch in your abdomen and arch your upper back, stretching your head and neck back. Take 3–5 slow rhythmical breaths and then either release or continue to step 3. To release, inhale and engage your abdominals and buttock muscles to lift your chest back up.

3 Exhale as you reach back for your heels and keep pressing your chest and hips forward. Take your head back and look back. Hold for as long as you are comfortable and then inhale as you engage your thigh, buttock and abdominal muscles in order to come out of the pose. Relax in child's pose.

Related poses

Wheel (pages 126–7)

Diamond (page 134)

Hold for as long as you are comfortable.

Half spinal twist ARDHA MATSYENDRASANA

◆ GOOD FOR: Flexibility of the spine

This twist produces a lateral movement for the spine. It is a healing pose, toning and stretching the liver and kidneys as the digestive fire is made strong and the large intestine is massaged, while flexibility and tone are brought to the back. Practise first with one leg straight and then, once your spine gains some flexibility to rotate, practise with the bottom leg bent.

Hold each pose as instructed.

Half twist with straight leg

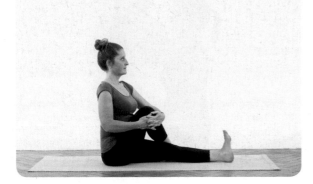

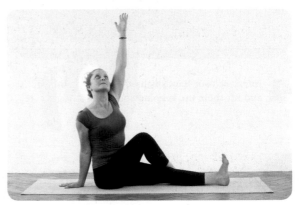

1 Sit with your legs stretched in front of you. Bend your right leg and cross it over the left, placing the foot flat on the floor. Pull your right knee close into your body and keep your spine and head lifted and in a straight line.

2 Place your right hand on the ground behind your back. Inhale as your raise your left arm, lifting all the way out of the left hip.

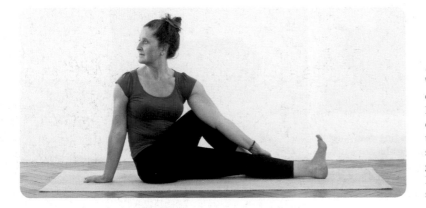

3 Exhale as you bring the back of your left arm against the outside edge of your right thigh. Bring your left hand to the outside edge of your left leg. Turn your head to look over and above your right shoulder. Your right thigh should gently press against the abdomen. Hold for 1 minute and then repeat steps 1–3 on the other side.

Half twist with bent legs

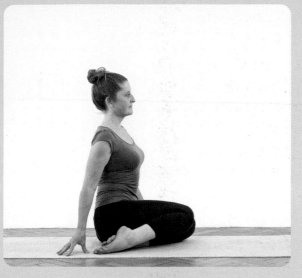

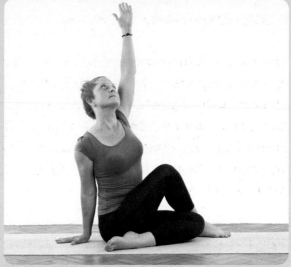

1 From a kneeling position shift your weight to the left so you are sitting with your hips next to your feet.

2 Place your right hand on the ground behind your back. Cross your right foot over your left thigh. Inhale and raise your left arm, looking up.

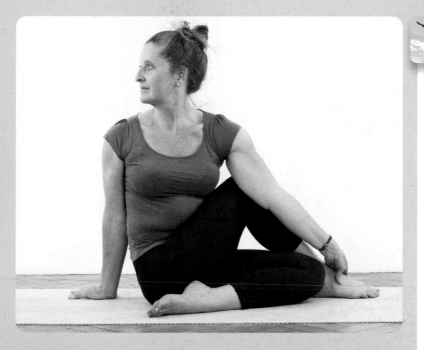

guru guide

• Focus on lifting and lengthening your spine and then twisting.

• ADVANCED HAND POSITION: to further open in the twist, take your back hand around your waist and bring your front arm under your lifted leg. Take hold of the back hand.

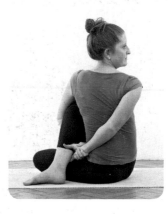

3 Exhale as you bring the back of your left arm against your right leg. Try to get the back of your shoulder close to the outside edge of your knee. Hold onto the inside edge of your right foot with your left hand. Turn your head and look over your right shoulder. Hold for 1–2 minutes and then repeat steps 1–3 on the other side.

Tiptoe balancing twist

◆ GOOD FOR: Strengthening your feet and mobilizing your toes

Balancing on tiptoes improves the flexibility in the ankles and knees, preparing the legs for the meditation poses. The twist also works on lateral flexibility in the spine and brings a gentle massage to the internal organs as well as developing balance. Start by practising steps 1 and 2, then work with step 3.

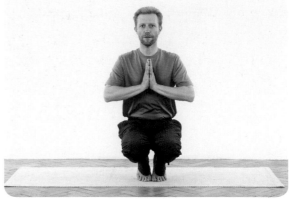

1 From kneeling, tuck your toes under your body with your feet together and come into a balancing position. Bring your hands into prayer position. Let your hips touch your heels, keep your spine straight and thighs together. Focus your gaze point straight ahead and take 2 breaths.

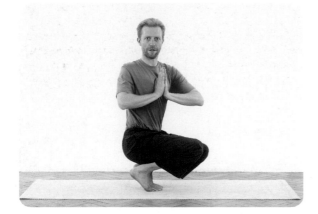

2 On an exhalation, twist your body around to the right, then inhale and come back to the centre and exhale over to the left side. Repeat 3 times on each side, moving with breath in a dynamic movement.

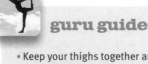

guru guide

• Keep your thighs together and hips down towards your heels. At the same time, concentrate on your focal point and keep your breath rhythmical.

Hold for 5 breaths and repeat on the other side.

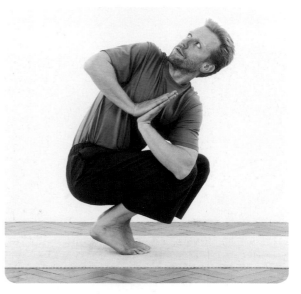

3 Start from centre (as in step 1) and, on an exhalation, twist your body to the right, bringing your left elbow against the outside edge of your right thigh. Keep your elbows in a straight line and bring your hands to the centre of your chest. Look up. Hold for 5 breaths and repeat on the other side.

Squat twist

◆ GOOD FOR: Strengthening your ankles

Related pose
Crow (pages 102–3)

This squat and twist boosts circulation in the legs and increases flexibility in the ankles, knees and hips as well as grounding the body. It is good preparation for the poses on pages 108–9.

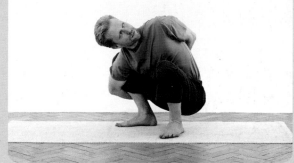

1 Squat with your feet slightly turned out and bring your hands together in prayer position. Press your elbows gently against the inside of your knees as you allow your hips to sink towards the ground. Keep your head lifted. Hold this for 5 breaths and focus on your legs and hips.

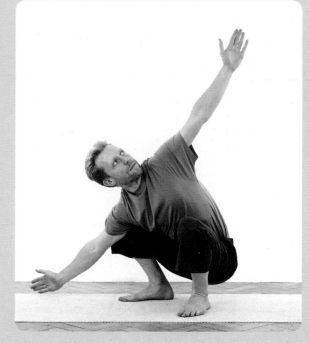

2 On an exhalation stretch your arms wide, pressing the back of your lower arm against the inside of your leg. Look up to your raised arm. Hold for 5 breaths. Return to step 1 and repeat on the other side or continue to step 3.

3 Exhale as you wrap your right arm around your right thigh and bring your left arm around your back. Clasp your hands (see below), twist the chest open and look up. Hold for 5 breaths and repeat on the other side.

Hold the pose for 5 breaths.

guru guide

• Keep your feet flat on the floor; drop your hips down and keep your chest lifted. Focus on your hip and opening up your chest.

• When clasping your hands behind your back in step 3, use the hold shown right.

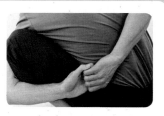

Tree VRKSASANA

◆ GOOD FOR: Strengthening your feet, ankles and legs

All balancing poses are about finding our roots, connecting to the earth and then letting the pose grow from a firm connection to our foundations. Practising these poses promotes physical, mental and emotional poise. They teach us to work with gravity and bring lightness in body and mind.

Vrksa means 'tree' and in this pose the standing leg needs to be strong and root down so the rest of the body can be light and elongate upwards, like the branches of a tree, reaching to the sky.

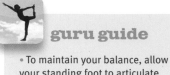

guru guide

• To maintain your balance, allow your standing foot to articulate its connection to the ground.

Related pose

Knee to chest balance
(page 59)

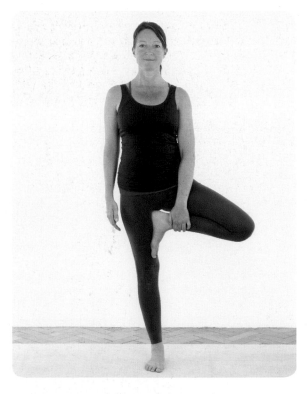

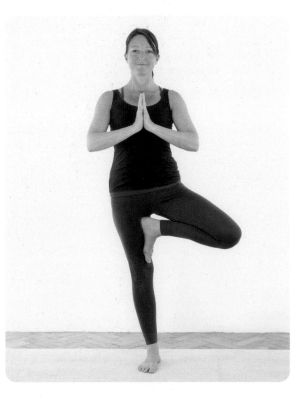

1 Stand centred and straight. Steady your breath and fix your gaze point. Bring the sole of your left foot to the inside of your right thigh. Press the foot to the thigh and thigh to the foot to activate an upward lift.

2 Bring your palms to prayer position in the centre of your chest. Keep your breath rhythmical and steady your balance, holding for 5–6 breaths.

Hold each part of each pose as instructed.

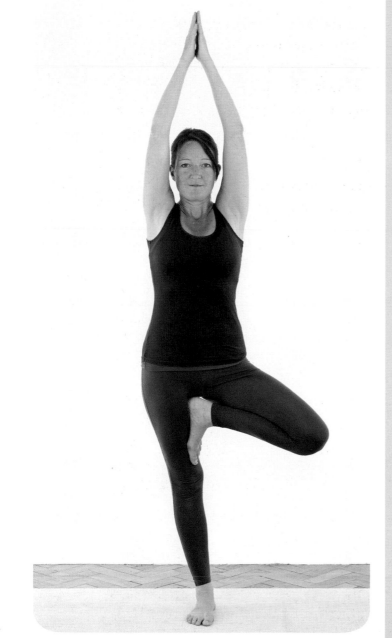

3 Inhale and raise your arms above your head. Keep your shoulders relaxed and stretch your arms straight. Hold for as long as you can and then repeat steps 1–3 on the other leg.

Working in the pose

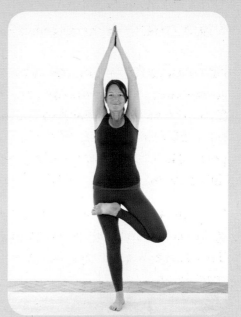

Hold the back of your left foot in your right hand and place it as close to your right hip as you can. Press the top of the foot against the thigh. Bring your palms to prayer position and inhale as you raise your arms. Swap legs.

To challenge the balance further, close your eyes. For an arm variation, open your arms wide like the branches of a tree and bring your hands into *chin mudra*. Swap legs.

Crow KAKASANA

◆ GOOD FOR: Developing balance, coordination and strength

Kaka is a crow and this balancing pose resembles a bird as the arms become its legs and the body is lifted away from the floor giving you a sense of taking flight. It develops strength in the wrists, arms and shoulders.

Related pose
Side crow (page 136)

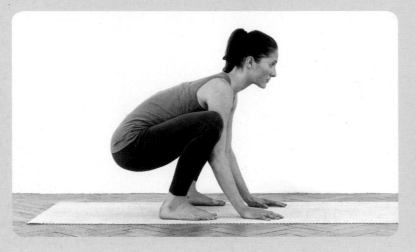

1 Squat on the floor and put your hands on the ground in front of you a shoulder-width apart and with your hands slightly turned in. Keep your arms slightly bent and place your knees around your upper arms.

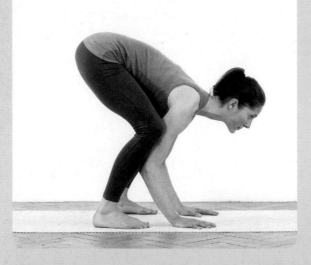

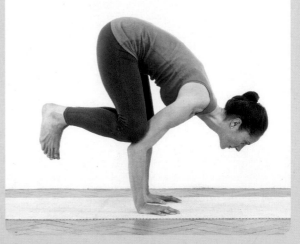

2 Lift your hips up high, securing your knees around your upper arms. Fix your gaze point straight ahead. Start to shift your weight forward into your hands. Keep your breathing deep and rhythmical.

3 Keep looking forward and shift the weight onto your hands as you lift your feet off the ground, holding your breath as you come into the pose. Hold the pose for a couple of breaths and then come back into step 2.

guru guide

• For the best hand and arm position, place your hands shoulder-width apart and spread your fingers wide. Lightly turn in your hands so your elbows can bend towards the side to support your knees.

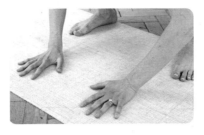

Hold for a **couple** of **breaths** and **build up** to 30 seconds.

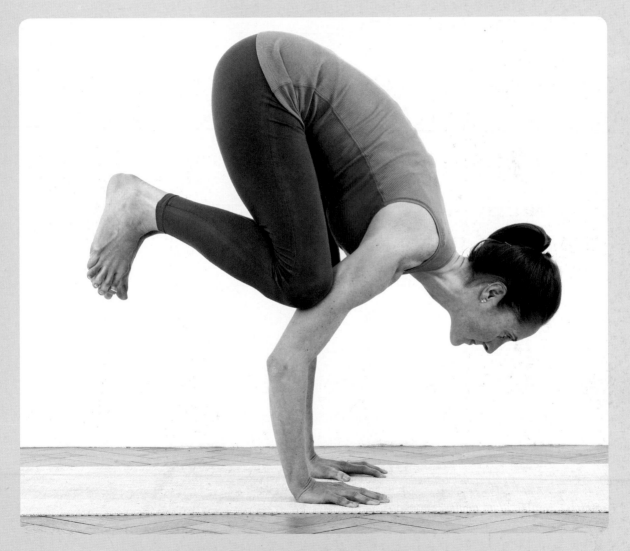

4 Once you feel confident with step 3, see if you can work on this devleopment of crow. Inhale and straighten your arms as you lift your hips higher. Move the gaze of your eyes towards the floor, but keep looking forward. Hold the pose for a couple of breaths and build up to 30 seconds.

Hands to feet pose PADA HASTASANA

◆ GOOD FOR: Stretching your leg muscles and hamstrings

This pose offers a deep extending stretch for the leg muscles and hamstrings while giving an extension for the spine. *Pada* means 'foot', and *hasta* is a 'hand'. It gently increases blood supply to the brain and boosts mental alertness. The idea is to keep your legs straight and hinge from the hips. If you have very tight hamstrings, practise holding step 2 with your hands pressing into the wall. For this, you can have your feet hip-width apart.

guru guide

• Keep your legs straight to gain maximum stretch for the leg muscles and hamstrings.

• COMMON MISTAKES TO AVOID (see right): don't bend your legs or round your upper back because then your hips won't be properly aligned with your heels.

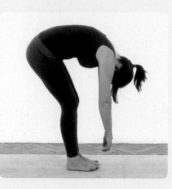

Alternative hand holds

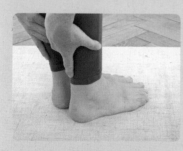

Wrap your hands around the back of your ankles with your thumbs on the outside. Focus on bringing your forearms behind your calves.

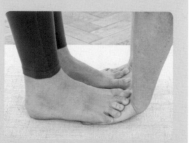

Place the palms of your hands under the soles of your feet. Hold for 1–2 minutes and then, on an inhale, return to standing.

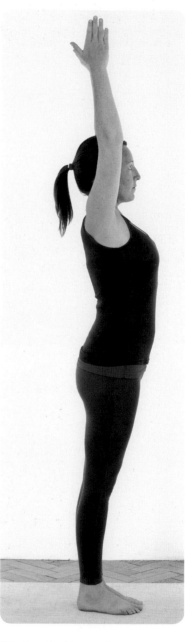

1 Stand with your feet together. Inhale and stretch your arms up over your head alongside your ears and with your palms facing forward.

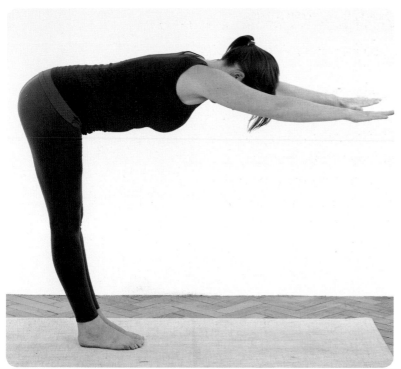

Hold for as long as you are comfortable.

2 Exhale, bending forward from your hips and keeping your back and arms in a straight line. Stay grounded in your feet with your weight evenly distributed, arches lifting and inner thighs together.

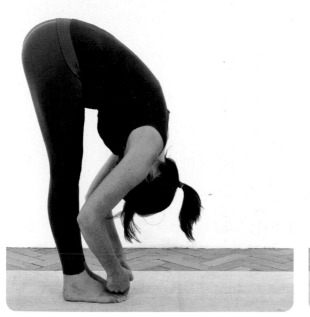

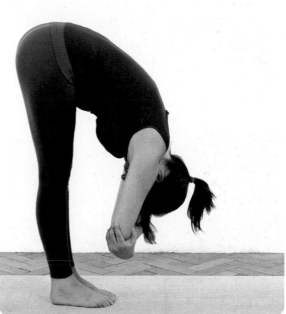

3 Continue to exhale as you fold your body all the way forward, taking hold of your big toes with your index fingers and drawing your chest in towards your thighs, head towards your knees. Hold for as long as you are comfortable and then return back up to step 1.

4 If your hands don't come down to the floor, hold onto the opposite elbow, framing your head in your hands. Keep your legs straight.

Triangle TRIKONASANA

◆ GOOD FOR: Toning the entire body

This standing pose and its variations are good for strengthening the legs, toning the waist and stretching the visceral muscles in the waist and spine. Practising them brings an awareness of alignment into the body and mentally brings a sense of direction and focus. They also teach us how to hold our mental course, breathing calmly and with focus through challenging situations.

Related poses

Head to toe pose (page 108)

Further standing poses (page 111)

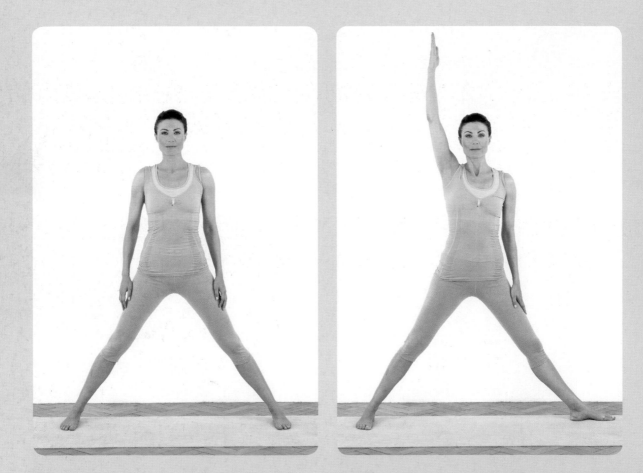

1 Stand with your feet about 90 cm (3 ft) apart. Keep the arches of your feet lifted, to bring strength and energy into your legs.

2 Turn your left foot out to the side and place your left hand on your left thigh. Inhale and stretch your right arm up alongside your right ear.

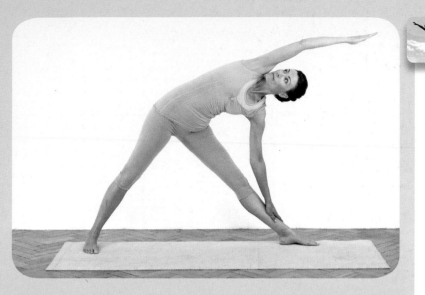

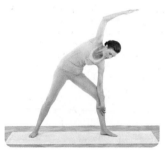

guru guide

• Keep your hips and shoulders aligned and your chest gently revolving up, with the chest open.

• COMMON MISTAKES TO AVOID (see below): don't look towards the floor, bend your front leg or lean forward with your legs too close together.

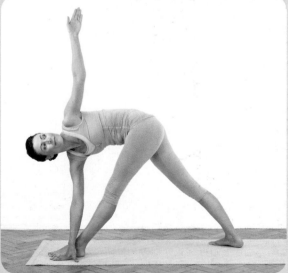

3 Exhale and bend your body over to the left, extending your right arm over the right ear. Make sure you do not lean forward or back, but keep your shoulders and hips in alignment. Reach for your left foot and extent your right arm over the ear, parallel to the floor. Turn your head and look up. Hold for 1 minute and then repeat steps 2 and 3 on the other side.

Reverse triangle

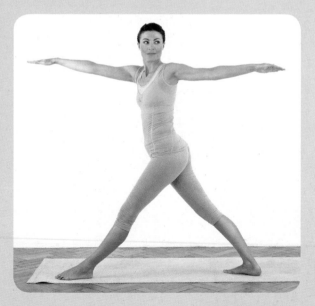

1 Stand with your feet about 90 cm (3 ft) apart, back foot turned out to the side and your front foot turned in. Turn your hips to face the front leg. Inhale and extend your arms out at shoulder height. Exhale and twist, moving your right hip forward and left hip back.

2 Continue to exhale as you bend forward, bringing your right hand to the outside edge of the left foot. If you can't reach the floor, place your hand on top of the foot or on your ankle. Stretch your left arm straight up and and look up. Hold for 1 minute and repeat on the other side.

Head to toe pose SIRANGUSTHASANA

◆ GOOD FOR: Strengthening your legs, especially your thigh muscles

In addition to strengthening the legs, standing poses open the hips, release stiffness from the shoulders and exercise the chest and lungs. They encourage deep breathing and are energizing. The aim of this particular standing pose is to bring the head to the ground, forehead alongside the big toe: *sirsa* means 'head' and *angustha* is the 'big toe'. The Sanskrit name for the variation, opposite, is *parsvakonasana*: *parsva* means 'sideways' and *kona* means 'angle', which sums up what this standing pose is all about.

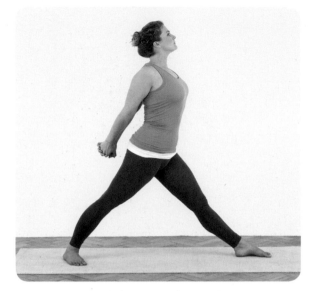

Hold each step of each pose as instructed.

1 Stand with your feet at least 90 cm (3 ft) apart. Turn your back foot all the way out, and turn your front foot slightly in. Turn your hips to face your front leg. Clasp your hands behind your back. Inhale, expanding your chest and look up.

guru guide

• Keep your feet grounded and the arches of your feet lifted.

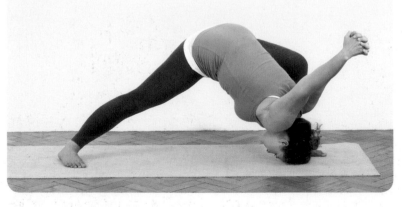

2 Exhale and bend your front leg, bring your head to the floor and stretch your arms away from your body over your head. Keep your back foot rooted on the ground. Hold for 1 minute and then repeat on the other side.

Related poses

Warrior (page 110)

Further standing poses (page 111)

Triangle (pages 106–7)

Developing the head to toe pose

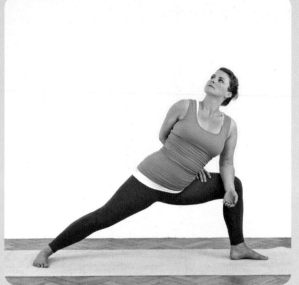

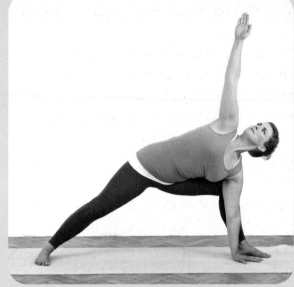

1 Stand with your legs wide apart and turn your left foot out to the side. Exhale as you bend your left leg, bringing the thigh parallel to the ground. Rest your left elbow on the left thigh and take your right hand around your back onto the left thigh. Keep your right hip lifted away from the left side and the chest open. Hold for 6 breaths and then release and repeat on the other side or continue to step 2.

2 Exhale and take your left hand to the ground inside your left foot and stretch your right arm straight up. Keep your back leg strong and look up at the extended arm. Hold for up to 1 minute and then either continue to step 3 or inhale, straighten the legs and release.

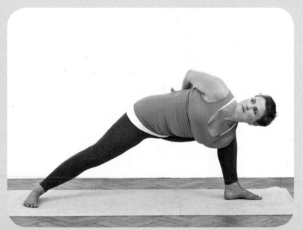

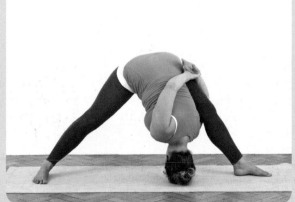

3 Take your left arm under the left leg and right arm around the back of your body. Hold onto the left wrist with the right hand, or clasp the hands. Rotate your chest up and back in line with your legs. Hold for 6 breaths and then continue to step 4.

4 Exhale as you straighten your left leg and fold your chest forward with the crown of your head pointing towards the floor. Hold for 6 breaths and then bend the front leg, release your hand, inhale and come up. Repeat steps 1–4 on the other side.

Warrior VIRABHADRASANA 1, 2, 3

◆ GOOD FOR: Strengthening your legs, especially your thigh muscles

These standing poses foster mental determination and focus, and develop balance. You can practise each pose separately from the basic warrior 1 standing posture, repeating on each side, or run them one into the next and then repeat the whole sequence on the other side.

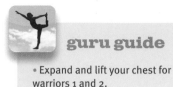

guru guide

• Expand and lift your chest for warriors 1 and 2.

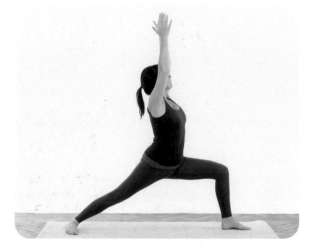

Related poses

Head-to-toe pose (pages 108–9)

Further standing poses (page 111)

Standing crane balance (page 142)

1 For warrior 1, stand with your feet wide apart. Turn your back foot out by 90 degrees and your front foot slightly in. Turn your hips to face the front leg. Inhale and raise your arms. Exhale as you bend your front leg, bringing your thigh parallel to the floor. Hold for up to 1 minute. Repeat on the other side or move to warrior 2.

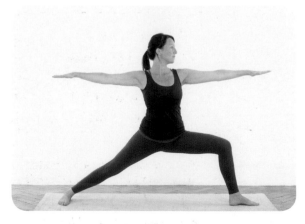

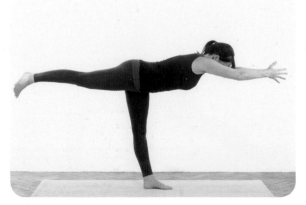

2 For warrior 2, exhale and bring your arms wide and parallel to the floor. Open your hips and chest to the side and look at your front hand. Hold for up to 1 minute. Repeat on the other side or move to warrior 3.

3 For warrior 3, inhale and lift your arms over your head, turning your hips forward. Exhale and lean over your left leg. Inhaling, lift the right leg and straighten the left, parallel to the floor. Hold for up to 1 minute. Repeat on the other side or return to warrior 1.

Further standing poses

◆ GOOD FOR: Strengthening your legs

These standing poses give a gentle inversion to the upper body stimulating circulation and the flow of oxygen-rich blood to the skull and brain. This makes these standing poses calming and restorative as well as energizing.

guru guide

• Keep your hips square and feet grounded and focus on keeping your waist long and chest open.

Sideways extension

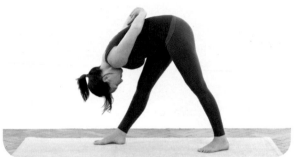 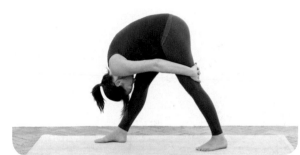

1 Stand with your feet apart and as for warrior, opposite. Bring your palms into prayer position behind your back, lifting your elbows. Inhale and lift your chest, then exhale and bend forward. Hold for up to 1 minute. Inhale, come up and repeat on the other side or move to step 2.

2 Reach back and hold around the back leg, bringing your chest closer to your front leg. Focus on your balance and rhythmical breathing. Hold for 6–8 breaths. Release your hands, inhale and stand up to come out of the pose. Repeat steps 1 and 2 on the other side.

Wide leg forward bend

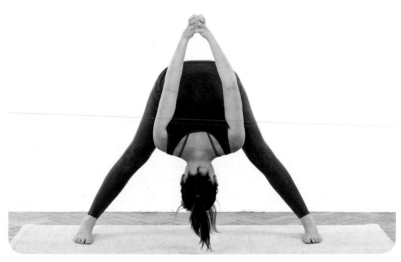

> *Related poses*
>
> Head-to-toe pose (pages 108–9)
>
> Triangle (pages 106–7)
>
> Warrior (page 110)

1 Have your legs wide apart with your feet parallel to the edge of the mat. Interlace your hands behind you. Inhale and open your chest, look up and exhale as you fold from the hips and bring your chest forward, crown of the head pointing towards the floor and arms extended over the back of your body. Hold for 6 breaths, inhale and come back up.

Headstand preparation

◆ GOOD FOR: Building strength

Out of all the hundreds of asanas and their variations, headstand is considered the king of asanas. It is a powerful pose, in which the whole body is inverted. It stimulates the crown of the head, awakening the higher energy centres in the body. Headstand not only builds tremendous strength and coordination in your body, it also tones the cardiovascular system and balances your nervous and glandular systems.

Reversing the normal pull of gravity in the body, blood is encouraged to flow to the skull and brain, so great relief is brought to the spine and all major joints in the body.

The full headstand is described on pages 116–17 following the dolphin, described here. This is a preparatory exercise and is helpful for all levels of practice as it develops shoulder, arm and upper body strength.

guru guide

• If you have high blood pressure or are recovering from a head or neck injury, avoid practising headstand.

• Keep your shoulders lifted away from your ears and try not to arch your back.

• Before practising headstand (pages 116–17) and the variations that follow on pages 118–19, spend a moment breathing and visualizing the pose.

The dolphin

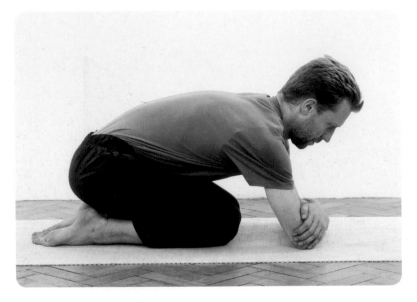

Related poses

Inverted V practices (pages 54–5)

Headstand (pages 116–17)

Headstand variations (pages 118–19)

1 Relax in child's pose before beginning (see page 30). Spend a moment breathing and visualizing the pose. Lift your head up from child's pose. Clasp your hands around the opposite arms, to get the correct measurement of the elbows, and then place your forearms on the floor.

Repeat the dolphin 4–10 times.

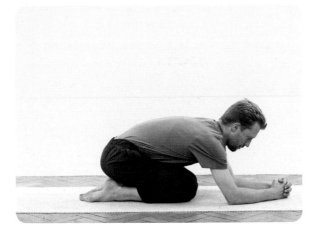

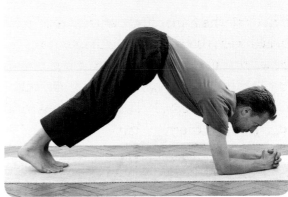

2 Interlace your hands and extend the forearms forward, and keep your palms open. The forearms and hands now form a tripod base for the headstand.

3 Tuck your toes under and inhale as you lift your hips, so the body makes an inverted 'V' shape. Keep your head up and look forward.

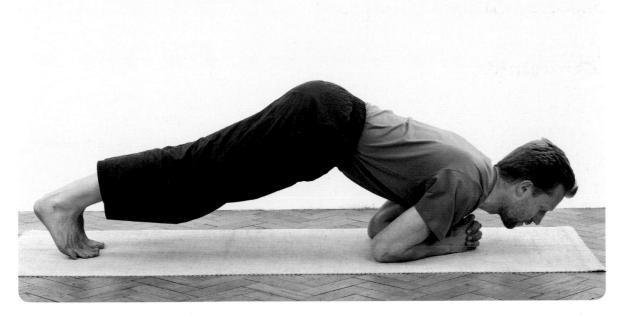

4 Exhale and move your body forward towards the floor. Keep your head and chin moving forward. Then inhale again, taking your hips up and back into the position shown in step 3. Once again on the exhale, move forward to step 4. Repeat 4–10 times. Rest in child's pose (see page 30).

Headstand SIRSASANA

◆ GOOD FOR: Developing concentration and balance

When starting, just practise steps 1–4, hold for a few breaths and then come down, either repeating or practising another round of dolphin (see pages 114–15). For guru guide advice, also see pages 114–15.

Related poses

Headstand preparation and variations (pages 114–15 and 118–19)

Scorpion (pages 120–1)

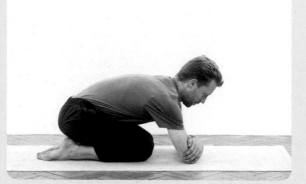

1 Lift your head up from child's pose. Clasp your hands around the opposite arms, to get the correct measurement of the elbows, and then place your forearms on the floor.

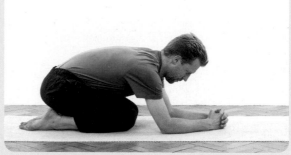

2 Interlace your hands and extend the forearms forward, keep the palms open. The forearms and hands now form a tripod base for the headstand.

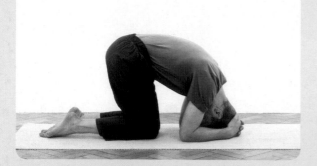

3 Place the crown of your head on the floor so it is gently supported in the cup of your hands. Press your forearms in the floor and keep your shoulder blades sliding down your back away from your ears.

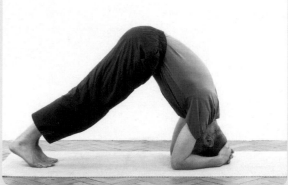

4 Tuck your toes under and lift up your hips. Take a few deep breaths.

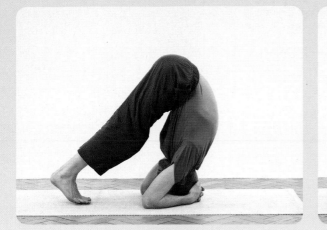

5 Walk your feet in as far as you can towards your head, lifting your hips so the back becomes straight. Keep lifting your shoulders and keep the base strong.

Hold for 30 seconds, building up to 5 minutes.

6 Using your abdominal and lower back muscles, draw your knees into your chest. If this is too difficult, try one leg at a time to begin with. Keep your knees into your chest while you stabilize and focus on the balance. Keep your knees and heals together and breath rhythmically.

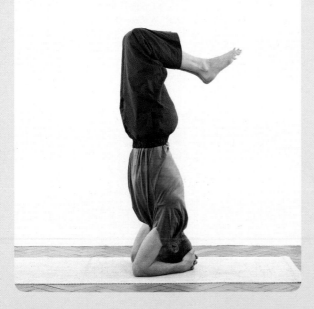

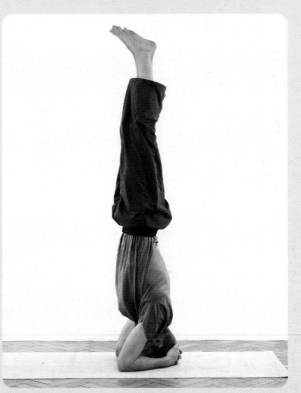

7 Slowly lift your thighs, keeping the knees bent. Focus on the balance by drawing your navel in towards your spine and pressing your forearms into the ground.

8 Extend your knees and straighten your legs. Keep your feet relaxed. Hold the pose for 30 seconds, breathing deeply, and build up to 5 minutes. Reverse down through steps 7–1. Rest in child's pose (see page 30).

Headstand variations

◆ GOOD FOR: Building confidence and spatial awareness

Once you have mastered headstand for 2 minutes, you may like to try some variations to further develop balance and concentration. Begin each of the following headstand variations from the basic headstand on page 117, step 8.

guru guide

• Keep breathing deeply and rhythmically to help you maintain your balance.

• Keep your shoulders away from your ears and take care not to arch your back.

Legs wide

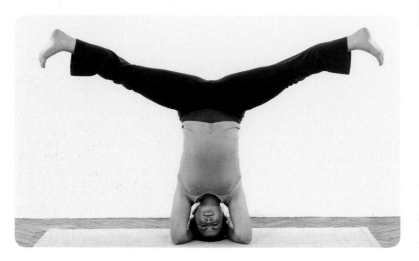

1 Exhale as you stretch your legs as far apart as you can, allowing gravity to stretch the legs towards the ground. Hold and breathe deeply for at least 8 full breaths.

Scissor legs

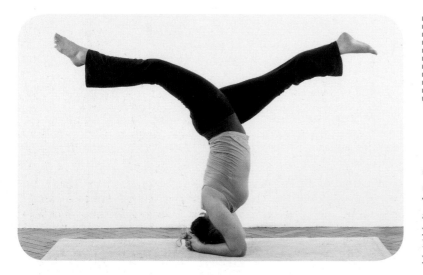

Related poses

Headstand preparation and headstand (pages 114–17)

Scorpion (pages 120–1)

1 Exhale and take your right leg forward and your left leg back. Try to move them to an equal distance apart, then change your legs. Once you feel balanced, try to work your legs back and forth, alternating with your breath.

Lower legs to the ground

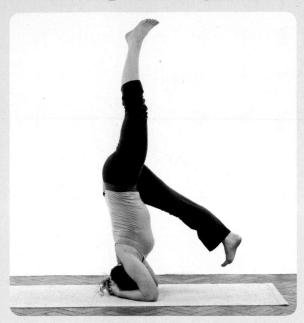

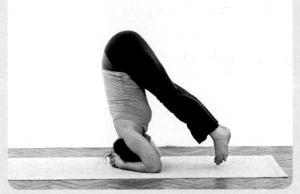

Repeat any of these **variations** a few times while in **headstand.**

1 Exhale and lower your right leg down as far as you can towards the floor. Keep your left leg lifted straight up. Inhale and raise your right leg back up. Repeat with your left leg. Keep your breathing rhythmical.

2 Once you have built up some control and strength lowering single legs towards the floor, exhale and lower both legs as far as you can. Keep your legs together. On the inhale bring your legs back up.

Lotus headstand with variations

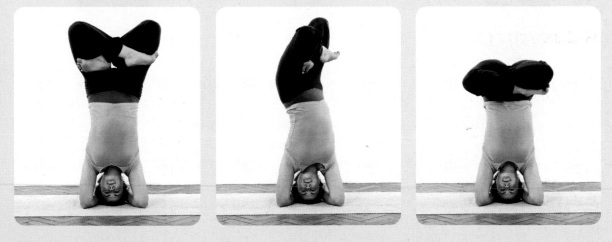

1 Exhale and bring your legs into lotus (see seated version on page 149). Keep your knees lifting up and thighs vertical. Hold the pose for a few deep breaths.

2 Exhale and twist your body to the side. Take 2 breaths and twist to the other side. Press your arms into the ground and breathe deeply and rhythmically.

3 Exhale and bend from the hips, bringing the tops of your thighs so they are vertical to the floor. Keep your back straight, inhale and lift your legs back up.

Scorpion VRISCHIKASAN

◆ GOOD FOR: Building confidence, concentration and balance

Scorpion requires strength, balance and a flexible spine. It is a harmonizing and calming inverted pose as the nervous system and glandular system are stimulated and balanced. It brings a deep stretch to the back muscles and increases blood flow to the brain. To prepare for scorpion, practise headstand for balance and wheel for flexibility.

Hold for as long as you are comfortable.

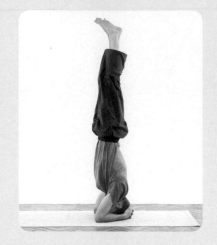

1 Start in headstand (see page 117), then exhale and start to arch your back. Bend your knees, and take your legs slightly apart.

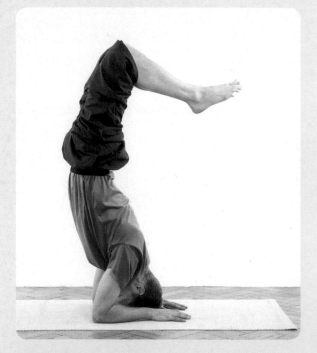

2 Begin to move your hips forward, then release the clasp of your hands and place your forearms and hands on the floor, shoulder-width apart. Press your forearms down into the ground and keep your shoulders lifted.

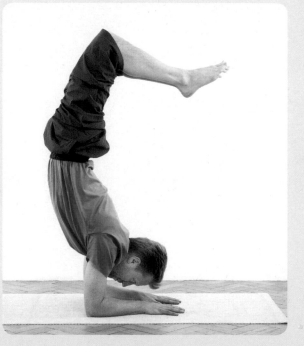

3 Lift your head and continue to arch your back. Keep your upper arms and forearms at a 90-degree angle.

• Keep your forearms parallel throughout to aid balance.

• Your upper arms should be vertical, forming 90 degrees with floor.

• Lift your shoulders and always look forward.

Related poses

Headstand (pages 116–17)

Headstand variations (pages 118–19)

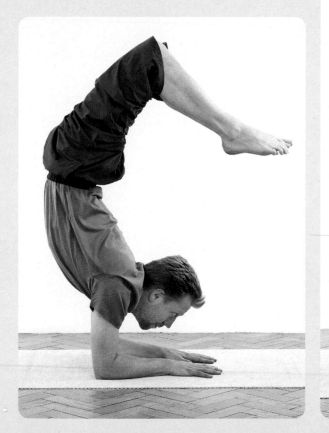

4 Look forward and bring your feet closer to your head. Exhale as you lower your legs even closer to your head, keeping your knees apart. Breathe rhythmically and hold the pose for several deep breaths.

5 Inhale and lift your legs into a more upright position. Keep your head lifted and hold for as long as you are comfortable. To come down, return to headstand: place your head on the ground, re-clasp your hands and straighten your body. Then follow steps 7–1 on pages 116–17.

advanced practices 121

Shoulderstand to bridge

◆ GOOD FOR: Developing back strength and flexibility

As you progress with the shoulderstand (see pages 68–9) and your back gets stronger, your body straightens with your feet aligned over your shoulders. This makes it easier to balance and explore some variations. Start with the full shoulderstand, *niralamba sarvangasana*. *Niralamba* means 'without support,' so this pose is literally a shoulderstand without support, where you are simply balancing on your head, neck and shoulders. Then think about moving onto a combination of shoulderstand and bridge and, finally, working through some variations once in bridge.

guru guide

• Once you have completed the bridge variations, return to shoulder stand, take at least 6 breaths before finally coming down to relax in corpse pose (page 31).

Full shoulderstand

Related poses

Bridge (page 48)

Shoulderstand (pages 68–9)

Fish (pages 72–3)

Wheel (pages 126–7)

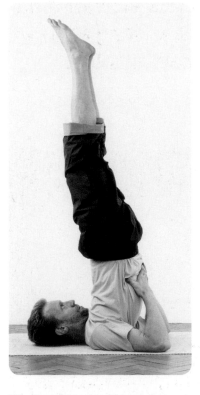

1 Start from shoulderstand, step 4 on page 69.

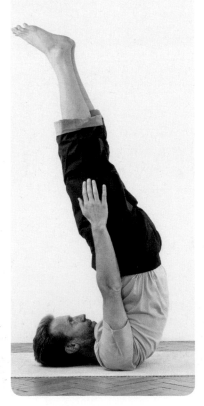

2 Once you feel balanced on your shoulders, extend one arm at a time along the sides of your body. Breathe rhythmically and hold for as long as you feel able. As you progress, you can hold this variation for several minutes. Re-support your back and either move out of the shoulderstand or prepare for another variation.

Shoulderstand to bridge cycle

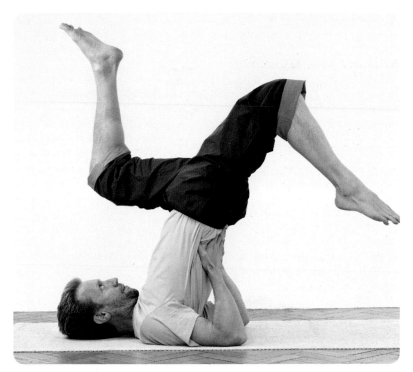

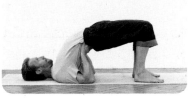

2 Keeping your hips lifted, bring your legs down to the mat, one at a time. Draw in your elbows and lift your hips. Keep your feet parallel and hip-width apart. On an inhalation, lift into shoulderstand. Repeat with the other leg.

1 Start in shoulderstand, as opposite. Keep the back of your rib cage lifting towards your heart and your heart lifting towards your chin. With your hands supporting your back, exhale and extend one leg forward, bending your knees, as you simultaneously bend your other leg back towards your head. This works as a counterbalance.

Hold each variation for as long as you are comfortable.

Working in the pose

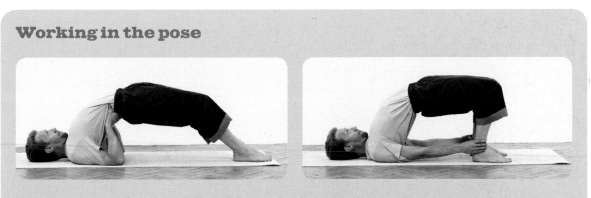

From the bridge walk your feet away from your body, then bring your feet together and work your legs straight. Keep your hips lifted. Hold and breathe for up to 1 minute, then walk your feet back. Either lower your body (see page 48) or continue with the next variation.

From the bridge walk your feet back towards your body. Keep your feet flat, reach forward and hold onto your ankles. Inhale and lift your hips. Hold and breathe for at least 6 breaths. Let go of your ankles and exhale as you slowly lower your back down onto the floor.

Tortoise KURMASANA

◆ GOOD FOR: Quietening your mind and senses

This forward bend requires flexibility in the hips, spine and legs and practising it tones the abdominal organs and increases circulation in the spine. It soothes the nerves and brings a state of mental relaxation. *Kurma* means 'tortoise' and this pose resembles the tortoise's shell, with legs and head protruding from under its shell.

guru guide

• Tortoise induces a peaceful mental state and releases anger and frustration, giving you the ability to surrender.

Related poses

Seated forward bends (pages 74–9)

1 Sit with your legs apart and bend your knees, keeping your feet flat on the floor. Bend forward and stretch your arms as far as you can under your legs with palms facing down.

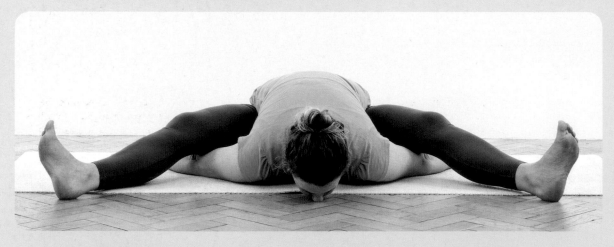

2 Exhale and straighten your legs and arms, bringing your chest and head to the floor. Press forward through your heels. Stay in the pose for as long as you can. To come out, bend your knees, slide out your arms, inhale and sit up.

Lifted leg forward bends

◆ GOOD FOR: Giving an extra stretch to your leg muscles

As well as stretching your leg muscles thoroughly, these forward bends develop balance and strength and tone the abdominal organs.

Related poses

Seated forward bends (pages 74–9)

Single leg forward bend

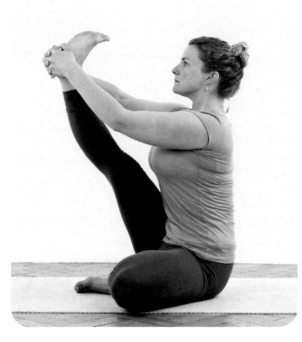

1 Sit with your legs stretched out. Bend your left leg and tuck in your foot. Bend forward and take hold of your right leg. Inhale as you lift the leg and take hold of your foot, ankle or leg. Exhale and pull your leg as close as you can towards you, keeping your spine straight. Hold for at least 6 breaths and repeat on the other side.

Balanced forward bend

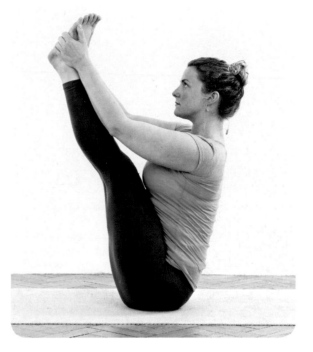

1 Bend your knees towards your chest and hold the soles of your feet. Exhale as you straighten your legs and pull them back towards your body. Keep your back straight and lift your gaze towards your toes. Hold for up to a minute and then release, bending your knees and placing your feet back on the floor.

Hold each pose as instructed.

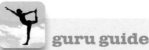

guru guide

• Keep your back straight and stretch your elbows to the side.

advanced practices 125

Wheel CHAKRASANA

◆ GOOD FOR: Freeing your spine

In this ultimate back bend all the energy centres in the body are stimulated as your body forms the shape of a wheel. This joyful, playful *asana* is a symbol of wholeness and, as such, the pose works on the respiratory, nervous, glandular, digestive and cardiovascular systems. The pose requires both strength and flexibility and gives you a greater sense of spatial awareness.

guru guide

• Straighten your legs as much as possible and lift up your navel.

• Keep your feet parallel, but be careful not to turn them out.

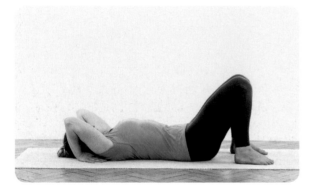

1 Lie on your back with your knees bent. Place your feet hip-width apart and have your heels under your knees. Place your hands on the floor alongside your ears with your fingers facing your shoulders.

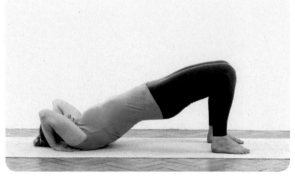

2 Inhale and press your hands and feet firmly into the ground and lift up your hips and back.

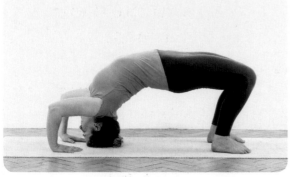

3 Continue to inhale as you lift your head and gently place it on the ground. Keep your elbows shoulder-width apart and pointing backwards. Hold and take a breath as you prepare to move on.

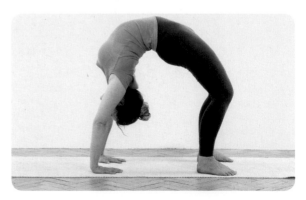

4 Inhale and straighten your arms and legs as much as possible and lift up your body. Gaze straight back and relax your neck. Hold the pose and breathe for several full deep breaths.

Working in the pose

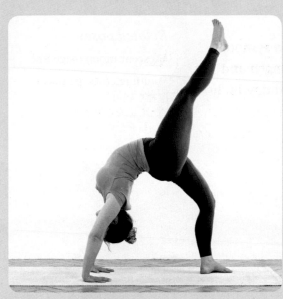

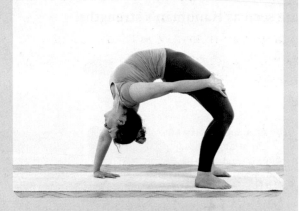

In the wheel, ground your balance into one foot and on an inhalation, lift up your other leg. Keep pressing your body away from the ground. Exhale and lower your leg and repeat on the other side.

In the wheel, ground your balance into one arm and on an inhalation, lift up your other arm. Reach your hand forward and place it on your thigh. Exhale and lower your arm and repeat on the other side.

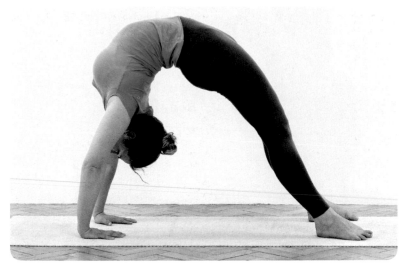

Hold for **as long as** you are **comfortable** and **repeat** up to **3 times.**

5 To straighten your legs further, move your torso towards your arms. Hold for as long as you are comfortable and repeat up to 3 times. To come out of the pose, slowly bend your arms, draw your chin towards your chest and lower your body back to the floor, reversing steps 2–1.

Related poses

Camel (page 93)

Shoulderstand to bridge (pages 122–3)

Full bow (page 135)

Diamond (page 134)

King cobra PURNA BHUJANGASANA

◆ GOOD FOR: Flexibility of your spine

King cobra is a complete back bend: *purna* means 'full' and *bhujangasana* means 'cobra'. As such, it exercises your neck, upper back and the whole of the spine. Lung capacity is increased as the chest expands and, in addition, the female reproductive organs are toned and adrenal gland function balanced.

guru guide

• Keep your knees apart, open your chest and lift your hips off the floor.

• Focus on lifting from your lower abdomen and creating space in your lower back.

• As you lift your chest, press your hands into the floor.

Related pose

Cobra (pages 84–5)

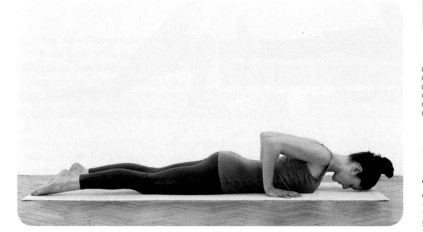

1 Lie on your abdomen. Place the palms of your hands flat on the floor in the centre of your rib cage towards your waist. Have your legs about hip-width apart and stretched back.

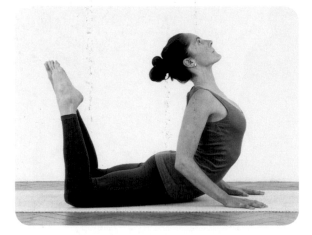

2 Inhale as you lift your head and chest and at the same time lift your lower legs off the floor. Bring your feet together and press your hands firmly into the ground to get a good lift in your chest. Take 1–2 breaths.

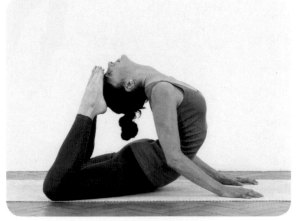

3 Inhale and lift your chest yet further. Exhale and take your head back and bring your feet to touch your head. Hold for a few deep breaths and release. Repeat up to 3 times. Relax in crocodile (see page 82).

Full locust PURNA SALABHASANA

◆ GOOD FOR: Strengthening your back and leg muscles

These advanced back bends require strength in the lower back, flexibility, full concentration and mental will power. They also give the benefits of inverted poses. For the locust and locust variations, see pages 86–9.

guru guide

• After each of these back bends, rest in child's pose (page 30).

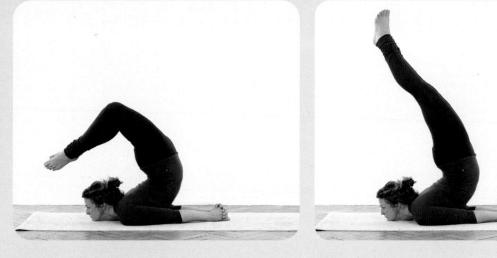

1 Lie on your abdomen, and take your hands and arms under the front of your body. Stretch your chin forward and extend your legs. On a deep inhale, press your arms into the ground and lift your legs all the way up.

2 Bend your knees and drop your feet towards your head. Hold for as long as you can, then either slowly roll down or inhale and lift your legs straight up. Hold for a few breaths and then exhale and come down.

Full locust variation

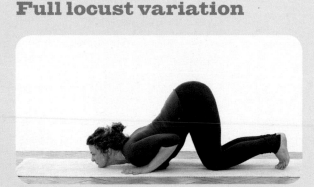

1 Kneel and bend forward, placing your hands on the ground, fingers in line with your shoulders and chin stretched forward on the floor. Elbows are bent and facing up. Support your weight with your hands and chin.

2 On an inhale and with one movement jump your legs up. Arch your back and let your feet come towards your head. To come out of the pose, slowly roll out. Relax in crocodile (see page 82).

Pigeon KAPOTASANA

◆ GOOD FOR: Deeply stretching your spine and leg muscles

Kapota means 'pigeon' and as the limbs of the body come together and the chest expands forward, this back bend resembles a puffed-out pigeon's breast. The pose brings a sense of lightness into the body and is very energizing.

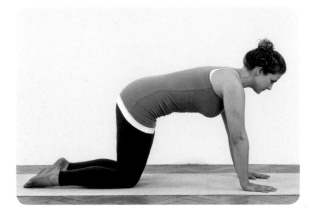

1 Come onto your hands and knees and take a couple of steady centring breaths.

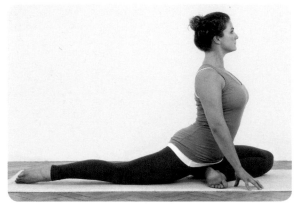

2 Draw your left leg forward and stretch your right leg back. Keep your hips facing forward and pelvis grounded. Keep your chest lifted.

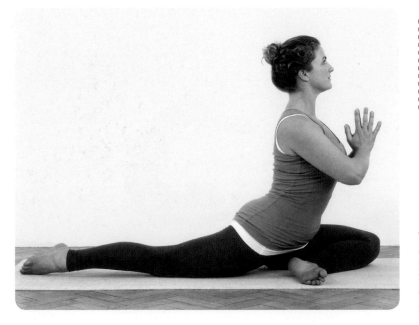

Related poses

Crescent moon (page 92)

Full bow (page 135)

Dancer (pages 140–1)

3 Once you feel steady, release your hands from the floor and bring them together in prayer position. Take several deep rhythmical breaths and either continue to step 3 or release and repeat the pose on the other side.

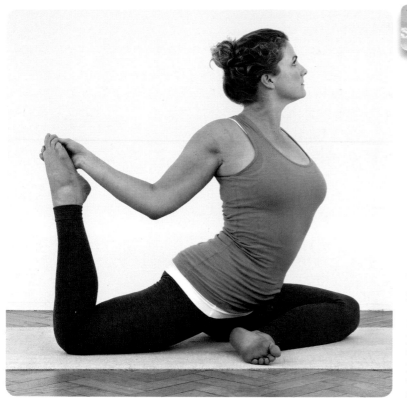

guru guide

• Gradually work your way through the steps of the practice, letting your breath guide you and don't force your body.

• Stay connected to the foundations of the pose, keeping your hips, buttocks and lower back down and expand the pose out of this grounded foundation.

4 Support your balance with your left hand on the ground. Bend your right leg, reach back and take hold of the inside edge of your foot. Keep your chest opening forward, lift your navel and point your sternum forward. Draw your left leg in towards your body. Take a few breaths and either release, repeating on the other side or continue onto the next step.

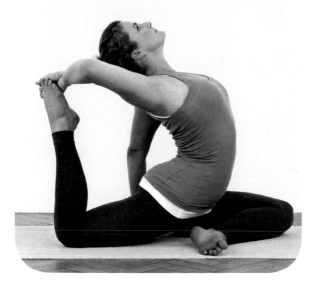

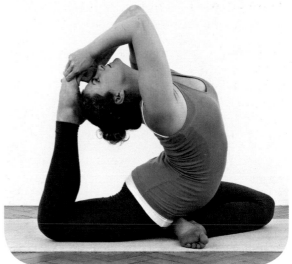

5 Exhale and turn your right arm so your elbow faces upwards and take your head back. Focus on the base of the pose as you stabilize and breathe.

6 Exhale and reach back with your left hand and take hold of the top of your right foot with both hands, drawing the foot in to touch the top of your head. Hold for as long as you can, keeping your breath rhythmical. Release and repeat on the other side.

advanced practices 133

Diamond PURNA SUPTA VAJRASANA

◆ GOOD FOR: Quietening your mind and senses

Poorna means 'full', *supta* is 'lying down' and *vajra* is a 'diamond', which accurately explains this deep back bend. It expands the thoracic spine and encourages deep breathing, strengthening your lungs and heart.

Related poses
Camel (page 93)
Wheel (pages 126–7)
Full bow (page 135)

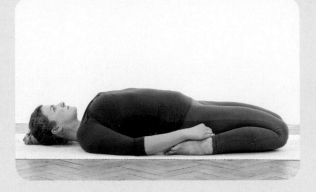

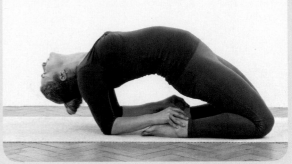

1 Start in a supine position with your buttocks on the ground between your heels. Keep your knees and thighs together. Place your hands on your heels. Focus on your breathing and expanding the front of the body.

2 Inhale and lift your hips and chest, pressing your thighs forward and dropping your head back. Support your body on your elbows and forearms and press the front of your lower legs firmly down.

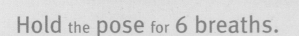

guru guide

• Make sure your knees stay close to each other.

• Keep your chest lifted and press your thighs forward.

3 Further arch your body and, exhaling, bring your head closer to the ground next to your feet. Hold the pose for 6 breaths. To come out of the posture, press your hands into the floor to lift your body. Rest in child's pose (see page 30).

Hold the pose for 6 breaths.

Full bow PURNA DHANURASANA

◆ GOOD FOR: Flexibility in your back, hips and shoulders

The full bow is a complete back bend and gives maximum stretch all along the spine. It is the natural progression from the bow described on pages 90–1.

Hold for as long as you are comfortable.

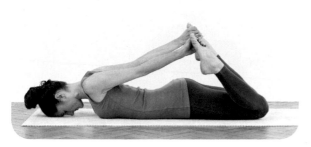

1 Lie on your abdomen. Bend your legs and reach back to take hold of the inside edge of your feet. To get a good hand hold, wrap your thumbs around your big toes (see the guru guide, below). Rest your forehead on the floor.

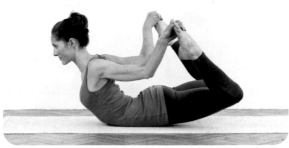

2 Inhale as you rotate your shoulders, drawing your elbows down and simultaneously lifting your head, and chest and thighs.

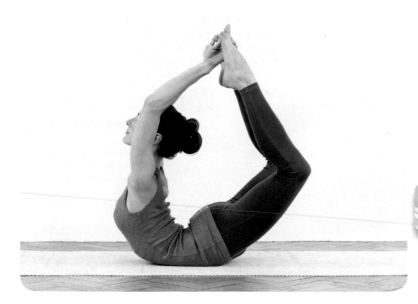

3 Continue to inhale as you lift your elbows out and up stretching your feet up and straightening your arms and legs as much as you can. Balance your body on your navel. Lift your head, look up and hold for a few breaths. Exhale as you gently lower your body and let go of your feet.

Related poses

Bow (pages 90–1)

Wheel (pages 126–7)

Pigeon (pages 132–3)

Dancer (pages 140–1)

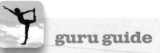

guru guide

• For the hand hold, wrap your thumbs around your big toes and fingers around the inside edge of the foot.

• Straighten your arms and legs as much as you can, extend your knees and look up.

Peacock MAYURASANA

◆ GOOD FOR: Developing mental and physical balance and strength

A challenging balance, this harmonizing pose resembles the plumage of a peacock and is a display of great strength and mental focus. It has a toning effect on the abdominal organs, massaging the digestive system and stoking the digestive fire aiding in the removal of toxins from the body. It also strengthens the arms and wrists.

> *Related poses*
>
> Side crow (page 136)
>
> Extended leg side crow twist (page 137)

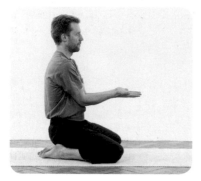

1 Kneel on the ground with your knees apart. Bring your elbows and hands together in front of your body, with your elbows in towards your abdomen.

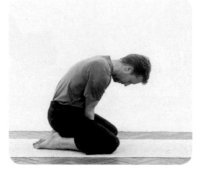

2 Put your palms on the floor fingers pointing to the back of the mat (see guru guide, below) and lean forward to rest on your arms. Keep your breath rhythmical.

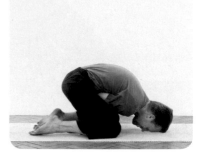

3 Lift your hips, bringing your forehead to the ground. Keep your elbows together and pressed against your abdomen.

guru guide

• Move your body forward to find your balance.

• When placing your hands on the mat, bring your wrists, elbows and forearms together, palms down and fingers pointing back.

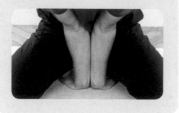

4 One at a time, extend your legs back, tucking your toes into the floor. Keep your legs straight and together and keep your arms strong, elbows together and abdominal muscles engaged.

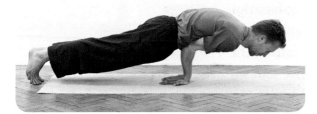

5 Inhale and lift your head and chest as you shift the weight of your body forward.

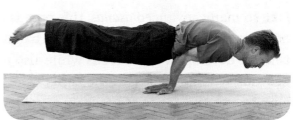

6 Take another breath, keep your elbows in and, as you inhale again, raise your legs. Keeping them together, hold the breath and, once you have the balance, continue to breathe, holding the balance for as long as you can. Release or try step 7.

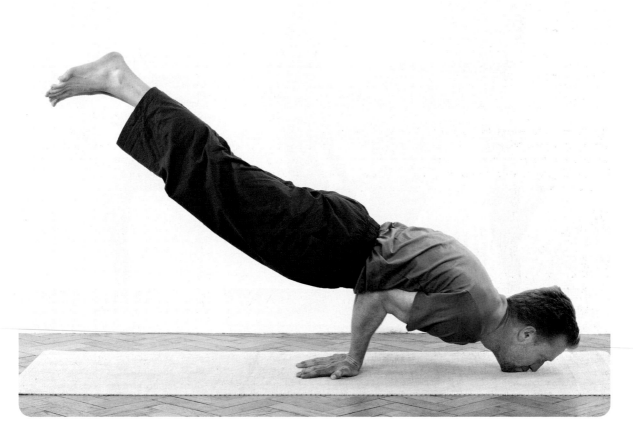

7 Exhale and slowly lower your chest towards the floor, chin towards the ground and lift your legs, keeping your body in a straight line. Hold for as long as you can and then release by lowering your legs to the ground.

The path to meditation

The last three steps of the classical eight-limbed yogic system of raja yoga (see page 15) concern meditation. The steps are *dharana* (concentration) and *dhyana* (meditation), which lead to the eighth and final step, *samadhi*, or super consciousness.

The *asanas* and *pranayama* practices covered in this book prime the body and mind ready for these higher rungs of raja yoga. Once you have some mastery of the poses and breathing practices, it is a natural progression to take the first steps in meditation. Meditation is the essence of all yoga practice – in the yoga sutras it is said that yoga is the stilling of the thinking mind.

An ancient universal system

Approaches to meditation vary, but the basic principles remain the same. The fruits of meditation are threefold – physical, mental and spiritual.

Physically, the heart rate and respiratory systems slow down. Every cell in our bodies is affected by our thoughts and emotions, so through nurturing positive thoughts and feelings in meditation, this has a harmonizing effect both at a cellular and energetic level. With greater mental focus, there is greater clarity. Clarity fosters purpose and direction, which creates emotional wellbeing.

Mentally, meditation asks us to look within, to turn attention to the inner world. For many, the vacillation of thoughts move this way and that, the mind is in a constant state of chatter, liking this, not liking that, grasping at things. This continual movement drains our ability to be still, to be present, to simply Be. The idea behind meditation is to gain control over this internal world, to find balance and peace.

Spiritually, meditation can lead to a greater sense of happiness, which is something everyone wants. If we try to find happiness in the shopping basket, in a relationship or in a certain job, we can be in an endless cycle of desire of if and when. However, with simple yoga and meditation techniques we all have access to the vast peace and happiness that is our true nature and lies within each one of us.

Meditation practice starts with concentration techniques (see pages 148–51). The source of all our actions is our thoughts and so they are the building blocks of our lives, to be sculpted as we choose. Thoughts have weight and power; they not only affect us, but also others and with loving, well-meaning thoughts you can send love and healing to others.

When first beginning to meditate, the mind may rebel, thinking up a hundred excuses why not to practise, but have patience and perseverance. Keep going with tenacity and regularity and success will be yours.

'Day after day let the Yogi practise harmony of soul: in a secret place, in deep solitude, master of his mind, hoping for nothing, desiring nothing.'

BHAGAVAD GITA 6 V 10

The first steps

For meditation, your body needs to be comfortable and your mind relaxed. Choose a time and place when you won't be disturbed. The best times to meditate are sunrise and sunset, but if these times don't suit you, the most important factor is to choose a regular time where you are free to practise undisturbed and feel calm. This will help you to form a positive habit. Choose a space that is clean and quiet. It can simply be a corner of a room that you set aside. Placing some flowers, a candle or an inspirational picture in this place can help set the mood and create a calm atmosphere.

guru guide

• *Tratak* (see below) strengthens your eyes, making them clear and bright. It also soothes the nerves and improves memory focus and concentration.

• Practise breath awareness in any situation. Try it while waiting for the bus or sitting at the traffic lights. It anchors us to the present moment and clears the mind.

Gazing with eyes open

Gazing at an object with unblinking eyes is known as the practice of *tratak*. It improves your mental focus and concentration in preparation for meditation. Start by practising for 5–10 minutes and, as your outer and inner gaze strengthens, build to 30 minutes.

Sit in a comfortable seated meditation pose (see opposite) and settle into steady rhythmical breathing. Focus on an object placed 60–90 cm (2–3 ft) in front of you at eye level. It could be a candle, an inspiring picture or an uplifting symbol. Focus your eyes without straining, gazing at the object for up to a minute. Then close your eyes as you continue to internally hold the image of the object.

Focus your internal gaze to the third eye, the space between your eyebrows. Keep your physical eyes relaxed as you focus the internal gaze. As the image starts to fade, open your eyes and re-focus on the external object.

Breath-awareness meditation

This form of meditation further develops concentration as you focus on your breath. Practise this meditation for 5 minutes.

Sit in a comfortable seated meditation pose (see opposite), with your hands in a *mudra* (see page 151). Keep your spine straight and eyes closed. Focus on your breath, watching it as it comes in and goes out. Notice the difference between inhalation and exhalation, in feeling, sensation and length. Breathe silently. Try to make the inhalation and exhalation equal in length, breathing in for a count of 4, then breathing out for a count of 4.

'Yoga pose is mastered by relaxation of effort, lessening the tendency for restless breathing.' **YOGA SUTRAS 2,51**

Meditation poses

Sitting for meditation is like doing mental housework. The mind is cleared of mental clutter and superfluous thoughts. It is a refreshing, energizing experience and has a physiological effect on your body and mind. The most important thing when you sit for meditation is that you are comfortable and breathe rhythmically. Your spine, neck and head should be straight, but not tense. Initially you may find it difficult to sit for any length of time without your back slumping or body tiring. With regular practice of both yoga postures and meditation, your body becomes more supple and back muscles strengthen, making sitting easier. The sitting positions on this page can be used for meditation. If your hips are stiff you may find it helpful to sit on a cushion or a folded blanket.

EASY POSE: SUKHASANA

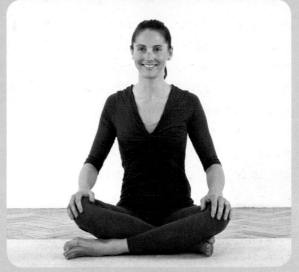

This easy-seated pose is a good one to start with for meditation practice. Cross your legs at the shins in front of you, relax your knees and connect your sitting bones to the floor. Keep your spine and head upright and straight.

HALF LOTUS: ARDHA PADMASANA

LOTUS: PADMASANA

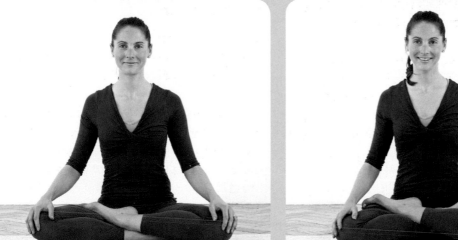

Sit on the floor, with your legs in front of you. First bend one leg and place your heel towards your groin. Bend your other leg, placing the back of the foot on top of the opposite thigh. Relax your knees towards the floor. When meditating try to change which leg you bring in first to equally open up your hips. This prepares you for the full lotus.

The lotus is considered to be one of the most important poses. Sitting on the floor, bend one leg and place the back of the foot on the opposite thigh. Then bring in your other foot and place it on the opposite thigh. Keep your knees down towards the mat.

Developing meditation

The quality of our thoughts colours the quality of our lives. When you first meditate, you might find it difficult to concentrate for long as your mind may not want to switch off, but be patient and persevere. Start by meditating for short lengths of time and you will soon build up to longer sessions. After practising the methods on the previous pages, try these two approaches.

guru guide

• If your mind wanders, bring it back to the practice. Work with patience and compassion.

• Try to practise in the same place and at the same time each day.

Sound meditation

Sound meditation develops awareness of listening without reacting. Practise each level of sound described here for 2 minutes.

Sit in a comfortable seated meditation pose (see page 149), with your eyes closed and your hands folded in your lap or resting on your knees in a *mudra* (see opposite). Turn your awareness to the experience of sound.

First listen to sounds in the furthest distance outside the building or place in which you are practising. Identify the sound and move on to the next one. Do not associate with the sounds or get involved with the story of any one sound. Just identify and observe.

Now move your focus to sounds in the middle distance, those in the building or the room. Move your focus from sound to sound.

Finally, move your awareness to the sounds that are closest to you, those within your own body, of your heart beating, of your blood pumping through your veins, of your breath. Spend a few minutes with this and then move on to listening to the silence that lies beyond these sounds.

Object meditation

Meditating on an object develops clear thinking and trains the mind to focus. Practise each level of meditation described here for 2–3 minutes.

Sit in a comfortable seated meditation pose (see page 149), with your hands folded in your lap or resting on your knees in a *mudra* (see opposite). Make sure that your breathing is steady and rhythmical and close your eyes in preparation.

Choose an object to focus on or a picture to explore. It could be a garden, so you could start by thinking of the grass, the moss, the flowers growing, the trees, birds and insects. Allow your mind to explore each aspect in as much detail as possible, but keeping it within the refines of the garden.

To challenge your mind further, just focus on one aspect of a garden, such as the flowers, and dwell on their colours and smells.

Then focus on just one plant or flower, visualizing it and concentrating on its details. Try to keep your mind within the refines of that one object.

Mudras (hand positions) for meditation

The word *mudra* means 'gesture' and they have a powerful psychological effect on the mind and body. First make sure your seated position is comfortable (see page 149) and then choose a hand position.

MUDRA OF CONSCIOUSNESS: CHIN MUDRA

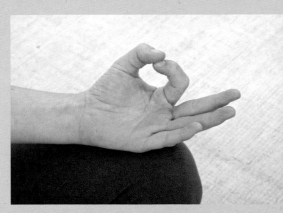

Fold the top of your forefinger under your thumb and place the back of your hands on the back of your knees. The other fingers remain extended but relaxed.

MUDRA OF KNOWLEDGE: GYANA MUDRA

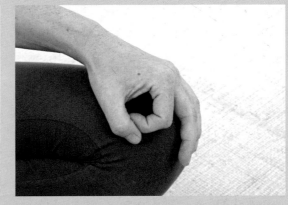

With your index finger under your thumbs, place your palms on your knees facing down. This is the same as *chin mudra*, but with your palms down.

MEDITATION MUDRA: DHYANA MUDRA

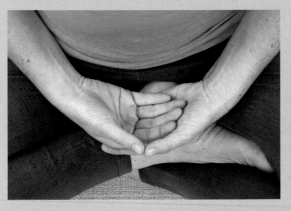

Place the palms of your hands in your lap, palms facing up, and right hand on top of the left with the tips of your thumbs touching.

CLASPED HANDS

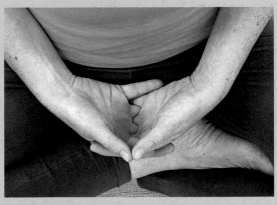

Interlace your fingers with your palms facing up and hands resting in your lap.

'Through processes of Yoga the body is rendered so subtle and pure that it is transformed.' HATHA YOGA PRADIPIKA

'Verily you are suspended like scales between your sorrow and your joy. Only when you are empty are you at standstill and balanced.'

KAHLIL GIBRAN

The power of visualization

The importance of proper relaxation cannot be stressed enough and is a must for developing concentration and practising meditation. In addition to the relaxation methods explained on pages 28–9, visualization reduces mental activity and nervous tension. Indeed, 10 minutes practising creative visualization can be as refreshing as several hours sleep.

Balancing visualization

Follow the complete relaxation practice on pages 28–9 and then, remaining in *savasana*, guide yourself through this visualization.

Start by focusing on your breath. Notice its rhythm, depth and any sensations that accompany the inhalation and exhalation. Allow it to become very subtle.

Move your internal focus to the base of your spine. Take three breaths and silently chant the mantra 'om' on your exhale. Make it long and give equal emphasis to the 'au' and 'm' sounds. Move your focus to your navel. Repeat the mantra on your exhalations and then three more times as you move your awareness to your third eye, the space between your eyebrows.

Visualize a line from the base of your spine to the crown of your head. On an inhalation move your awareness up to the crown, and on the exhalation move the awareness down to the base of your spine. Keep your awareness with your breath and continue to trace your breath up and down for 2–3 minutes.

Now direct your awareness to the base of your spine and become aware of your physicality, of the *earth* element within you. Focus on feeling grounded and on bringing this element into balance. Move your awareness to your lower abdomen, to the seat of the *water* element. Focus on its balance, your ability to be fluid and adapt like water. Move your awareness to your navel, the seat of *fire*, the creative force. Concentrate on the strength in this fire to digest and assimilate all that you need, for a strong physical and emotional constitution.

Take your focus into your heart centre and chest and become aware of the element of *air*. Focus on your ability to create and hold space within yourself. From here move your awareness to the space above the crown of your head, with your focus on the element of *ether*, your ability to have perfect balance in all aspects of your being through conscious thoughts and intentions, bringing all elements within you into perfect balance and harmony.

Conclude your practice by taking three conscious breaths, inhaling from the base of your spine to the crown of your head and exhaling back to the base of your spine. Focus on the balance and harmony within each aspect and element of your being.

Give yourself a stretch, sit up and come into a comfortable seated crossed leg position, chanting the mantra 'om' three times.

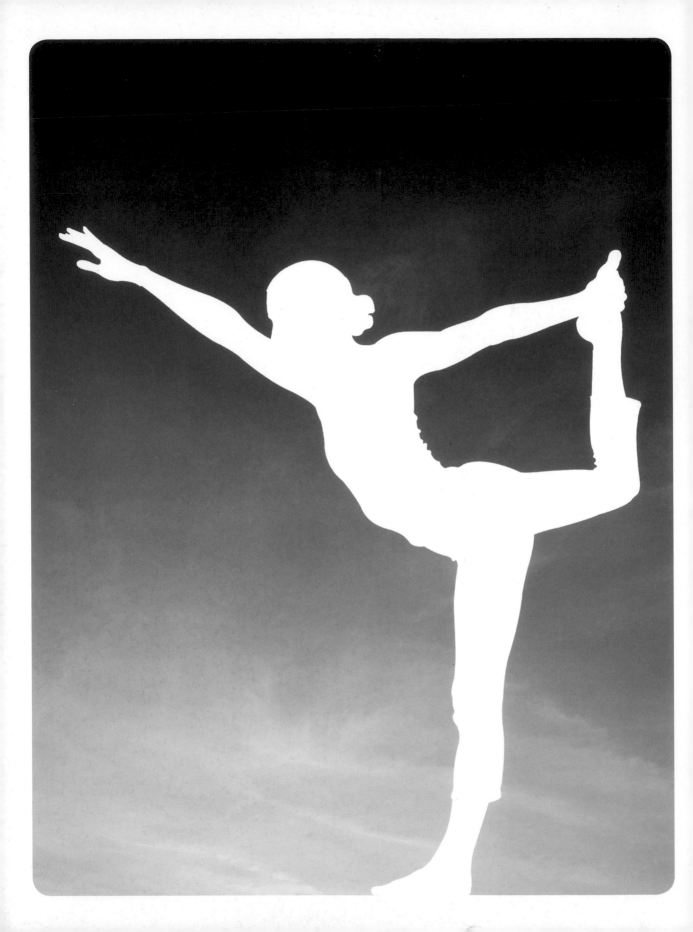

Yoga sessions

The sessions on the following pages use the poses
given in this book, combined in easy-to-follow routines.
There are sessions for beginners, intermediate and
advanced practitioners, to start your day, end your day
and give you an afternoon boost. They are designed to
systematically progress your practice, so repeat each set
of poses as many times as you like before moving onto
the next, progressing at your own pace.

Building a balanced practice

You don't have to be flexible to practise yoga, but practise and you will be. Whatever your age or level of fitness, you can benefit from yoga. Due to increased sedentary lifestyles many people suffer from backache and general stiffness. It doesn't matter how inflexible you think you are, with regular gentle stretching and breath work you will be amazed how quickly you can progress.

As you plan your sessions, include a selection of poses that feature a warm up, such as the sun salutation (see pages 63–7). Always finish with a final relaxation (see pages 28–9) and add some deep breathing exercises (see pages 26–7) and meditation (see pages 146–51) if time allows. Between the warm up and final relaxation, ensure you include poses from each of the areas shown on these pages.

guru guide

• If you have less time than suggested in the sessions on pages 158–71, you are better practising fewer poses and variations but doing them with focus. One pose done well is better than five rushed poses with a distracted mind.

Practise regularly and you will be amazed how quickly you can progress.

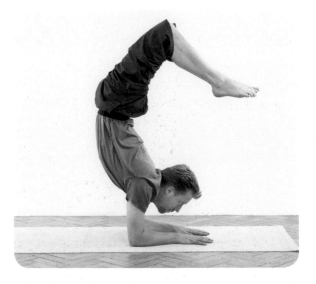

Inversions work directly on the heart. They improve blood circulation and calm the mind. By literally turning the body upside down, they let us see things from a new perspective. They also promote mental strength and develop willpower.

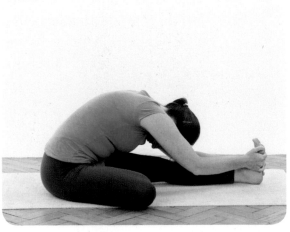

Forward bends have a calming effect on the nervous system. They massage the abdominal organs and relieve stiffness from the legs and back. Encouraging a reflective introverted state of mind, they are the opposite of backward bending asanas.

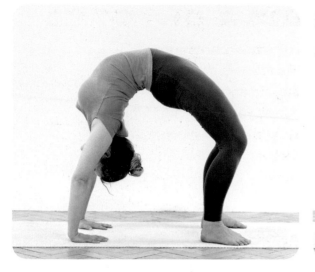

Back bends are extroverting poses. They open up our soft underbelly. They are bold poses that are energizing and give courage and help release fear of the unknown. They tone and strengthen the spine and stretch out the abdominal muscles.

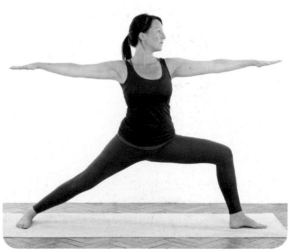

Twists are vital for spinal health. They increase the flexibility of the spine and bring energy into the navel region, which benefits digestion. Twists help untangle the knots of life that can get stuck in our stomachs and so also promote emotional health.

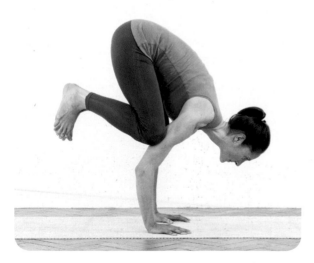

Balancing poses may be challenging if you lack balance in your lives. They call us to our centre and require focus and concentration. They promote physical and mental balance working with the forces of gravity.

Standing poses make your foundations strong. They strengthen your connection to the earth element and improve posture. They work on the leg muscles as well as those in the upper body to exercise the heart.

Beginner sessions 1

This series of practices teaches the breathing basics and concentrates on joint mobility. Keep your focus on bringing the movement and your breath together. It is important to take your time and not rush. To progress systematically, practise each sequence until you feel comfortable with all the poses. Ideally, start with the shortest session and practise it two to three times a week for two or three weeks and then move on incorporating what you can from the next sequence.

The **30-minute session** gives your body a gentle stretch and connects to your breathing. **The 45-minute session** works further on opening up the hips. **The 60-minute session** brings more of a focus to spine flexibility. Try to work through more repetitions of each exercise.

Start with 5 minutes relaxing in corpse pose (see page 31), then continue with your choice of routine and relax once more at the end in corpse pose for 10 minutes.

30-minute session

1 Abdominal breathing (page 24)

2 Eye exercises (pages 36–7)

3 Neck exercises (pages 38–9)

4 Shoulder exercises (pages 40–3)

5 Single leg raises (page 47)

6 Bridge (page 48)

7 Lying twist (page 49)

8 Mountain stretch (page 56)

45-minute session

1 Abdominal breathing (page 24)

2 Eye exercises (pages 36–7)

3 Neck exercises (pages 38–9)

4 Shoulder exercises (pages 40–3)

5 Foot exercises (page 44)

6 Butterfly (page 45)

7 Single leg raises (page 47)

8 Bridge (page 48)

9 Lying twist (page 49)

10 Stirring the pot (page 51)

11 Mountain stretch (page 56)

guru guide

• Make a commitment to yourself to finish the session once you have started it.

• Make the movements controlled and in rhythm with your breath, resting for as long as you need between poses using the relaxation poses on page 29.

60-minute session

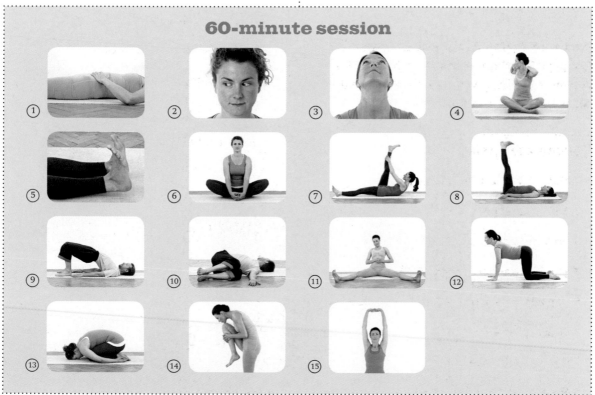

60-minute session

To progress systematically, practise each sequence until you feel comfortable with all the poses.

Beginner sessions 2

These sessions work with full yogic breath and prepare you for sun salutations. It is vital to master full yogic breath to progress with your practice, so as you work slowly through the sessions, concentrate on your breathing throughout. Rest as much as you need to between the poses and work to increase the number of repetitions from the beginner sessions 1.

The 30-minute session works mainly with spinal flexibility, stretching your hamstrings and opening your hips. **The 45-minute session** works on the whole body, particularly focusing on developing balance. **The 60-minute session** prepares you for sun salutation as well as strengthening your legs and promoting mobility in all your joints.

Start with 5 minutes relaxing in corpse pose (see page 31) and practise full yogic breathing (see page 25). Then continue with your choice of routine and relax once more at the end in corpse pose for 10 minutes.

30-minute session

1 Shoulder exercises 1 (pages 40–41)

2 Single and double leg raises (page 47)

3 Cat (page 52)

4 Tiger (page 53)

5 Bridge (page 48)

6 Butterfly (page 45)

7 Stirring the pot (page 51)

8 Seated spinal twist (page 50)

9 Dynamic energizing squats (page 58)

45-minute session

1 Neck exercises (pages 38–9)

2 Shoulder exercises 1 (pages 40–3)

3 Single and double leg raises (page 47)

4 Cat (page 52)

5 Tiger (page 53)

6 Bridge (page 48)

7 Butterfly (page 45)

8 Foot exercises (page 44)

9 Stirring the pot (page 51)

10 Seated spinal twist (page 50)

11 Dynamic energizing squats (page 58)

12 Knee to chest balance (page 59)

guru guide

• Work with your breathing and focus on keeping your foundations strong, whether they are your feet, hands or hips.

• Wait for two hours after a heavy meal before you practise and make sure you are warm enough as this helps your muscles work properly.

60-minute session

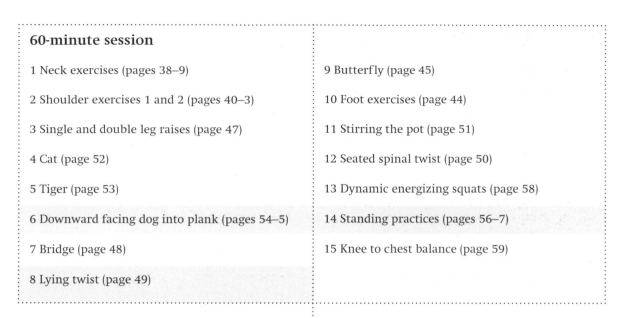

1 Neck exercises (pages 38–9)

2 Shoulder exercises 1 and 2 (pages 40–3)

3 Single and double leg raises (page 47)

4 Cat (page 52)

5 Tiger (page 53)

6 Downward facing dog into plank (pages 54–5)

7 Bridge (page 48)

8 Lying twist (page 49)

9 Butterfly (page 45)

10 Foot exercises (page 44)

11 Stirring the pot (page 51)

12 Seated spinal twist (page 50)

13 Dynamic energizing squats (page 58)

14 Standing practices (pages 56–7)

15 Knee to chest balance (page 59)

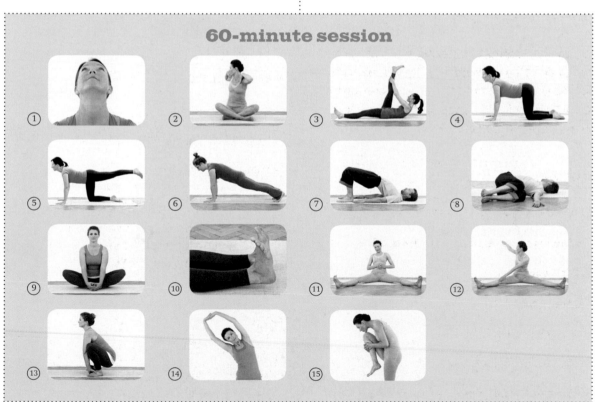

60-minute session

Rest as much as you need to between the poses.

Intermediate sessions 1

These sessions introduce sun salutation and all the elements of practice, building to a complete routine. In addition, the main breathing skills are introduced. Spend time on each session before progressing onto the next one. You will benefit from repetition, so don't be in a hurry to move on.

The 45-minute session works on stretching the back of your body, making your spine and legs flexible as well as learning the shoulderstand. **The 60-minute session** gives you a full but basic practice without any variations. **The 90-minute session** works with retention in alternate nostril breathing as well as working a little more deeply with your hips and forward bends.

Start with 5 minutes relaxing in corpse pose (see page 31), then continue with your choice of routine and relax once more at the end in corpse pose for 10 minutes.

45-minute session

1 Sun salutation (pages 64–7)

2 Leg exercises (pages 46–7)

3 Shoulderstand (pages 68–9)

4 Plough (pages 70–1)

5 Fish (pages 72–3)

6 Seated forward bend (pages 74–5)

7 Table top (page 81)

8 Half spinal twist with straight leg (page 96)

9 Hands to feet pose (pages 104–5)

60-minute session

1 Alternate nostril breathing without retention: 5 rounds (page 26)

2 Sun salutation (pages 64–7)

3 Leg exercises (pages 46–7)

4 Shoulderstand (pages 68–9)

5 Plough (pages 70–1)

6 Fish (pages 72–3)

7 Seated forward bend (pages 74–5)

8 Table top (page 81)

9 Cobra (pages 84–5)

10 Half spinal twist with straight leg (page 96)

11 Tree (pages 100–1)

12 Hands to feet pose (pages 104–5)

You will **benefit** from **repetition**, so don't be in a **hurry** to **move on.**

60-minute session

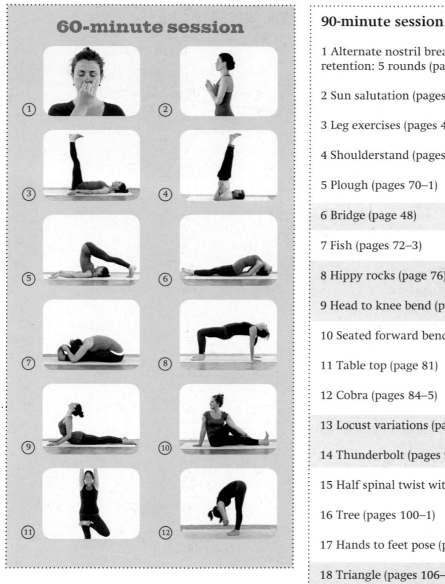

90-minute session

1 Alternate nostril breathing without retention: 5 rounds (page 26)

2 Sun salutation (pages 64–7)

3 Leg exercises (pages 46–7)

4 Shoulderstand (pages 68–9)

5 Plough (pages 70–1)

6 Bridge (page 48)

7 Fish (pages 72–3)

8 Hippy rocks (page 76)

9 Head to knee bend (page 77)

10 Seated forward bend (pages 74–5)

11 Table top (page 81)

12 Cobra (pages 84–5)

13 Locust variations (pages 88–9)

14 Thunderbolt (pages 94–5)

15 Half spinal twist with straight leg (page 96)

16 Tree (pages 100–1)

17 Hands to feet pose (pages 104–5)

18 Triangle (pages 106–7)

guru guide

• Gradually increase the number of rounds of sun salutation, starting with 3 and build up to 12 rounds. As you progress, hold each pose for longer.

• Relax between poses and keep focusing on your breath, always breathing in and out through your mouth.

• Pay attention to how you feel and the sensations within your body. Notice which poses challenge you more and try to spend a little more time on them.

• Make sure you focus particularly on the precision of your movement and positioning throughout.

Intermediate sessions 2

As you progress from intermediate sessions 1 to the groups of poses on these pages, focus on starting to hold the poses for longer and combining more of them to flow together before resting. For example, practise shoulderstand, plough and fish and then relax before continuing with the rest of the session.

The **45-minute session** concentrates on balancing and energizing all of your body. **The 60-minute session** then has more back bends and balances, challenging your focus and concentration. **The 90-minute session** includes pranayama practices and a full range of poses working on your flexibility and balance.

Start with 5 minutes relaxing in corpse pose (see page 31), then continue with your choice of routine and relax once more at the end in corpse pose for 10 minutes.

45-minute session

1 Sun salutation: 6 rounds (pages 64–7)

2 Leg exercises (pages 46–7)

3 Shoulderstand (pages 68–9)

4 Plough (pages 70–1)

5 Fish (pages 72–3)

6 Seated forward bend (pages 74–5)

7 Incline plane (pages 80–1)

8 Cobra (pages 84–5)

9 Tip toe balancing twist (page 98)

10 Hands to feet pose (pages 104–5)

60-minute session

1 Sun salutation: 8 rounds (pages 64–7)

2 Leg exercises (pages 46–7)

3 Shoulderstand (pages 68–9)

4 Plough (pages 70–1)

5 Fish (pages 72–3)

6 Seated forward bend (pages 74–5)

7 Incline plane (pages 80–1)

8 Cobra (pages 84–5)

9 Locust (pages 86–7)

10 Tip toe balancing twist (page 98)

11 Crow (pages 102–3)

12 Hands to feet pose (pages 104–5)

13 Warrior (page 110)

Focus on combining poses to flow together before resting.

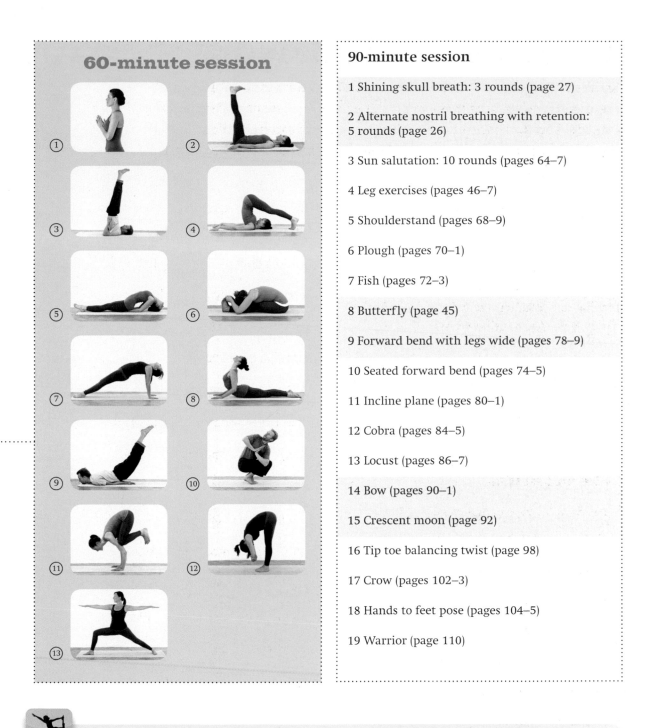

60-minute session

① ② ③ ④ ⑤ ⑥ ⑦ ⑧ ⑨ ⑩ ⑪ ⑫ ⑬

90-minute session

1 Shining skull breath: 3 rounds (page 27)

2 Alternate nostril breathing with retention: 5 rounds (page 26)

3 Sun salutation: 10 rounds (pages 64–7)

4 Leg exercises (pages 46–7)

5 Shoulderstand (pages 68–9)

6 Plough (pages 70–1)

7 Fish (pages 72–3)

8 Butterfly (page 45)

9 Forward bend with legs wide (pages 78–9)

10 Seated forward bend (pages 74–5)

11 Incline plane (pages 80–1)

12 Cobra (pages 84–5)

13 Locust (pages 86–7)

14 Bow (pages 90–1)

15 Crescent moon (page 92)

16 Tip toe balancing twist (page 98)

17 Crow (pages 102–3)

18 Hands to feet pose (pages 104–5)

19 Warrior (page 110)

guru guide

• Practise with your eyes closed, if you can, and feel the movement of energy within you.

• Hold the poses for longer and work to join them into a flowing sequence.

Advanced sessions 1

These sessions introduce the headstand and more advanced back bends. Focus on trying to hold the poses for even longer. Visualizing the poses will help you achieve them; believe that you can do them. Even if initially you don't get into the full posture, keep trying and eventually you will.

The 45-minute session works with the headstand, which is energizing and balances your nervous system. **The 60-minute session** includes more rounds of sun salutations to prepare your body for the advanced back bends. **The 90-minute session** then adds hip flexibility and balance as well as *pranayama* practices.

Start with 5 minutes relaxing in corpse pose (see page 31), then continue with your choice of routine and relax once more at the end in corpse pose for 10 minutes.

45-minute session

1 Sun salutation: 6 rounds (pages 64–7)

2 Leg exercises (pages 46–7)

3 Dolphin and headstand (pages 114–17)

4 Shoulderstand (pages 68–9)

5 Plough (pages 70–1)

6 Fish (pages 72–3)

7 Seated forward bend (pages 74–5)

8 Incline plane (pages 80–1)

9 Half spinal twist with bent legs (page 97)

10 Crow (pages 102–3)

11 Reverse triangle (page 107)

60-minute session

1 Sun salutation 10 rounds (pages 64–7)

2 Leg exercises (pages 46–7)

3 Dolphin and headstand (pages 114–17)

4 Shoulderstand (pages 68–9)

5 Plough (pages 70–1)

6 Shoulderstand to bridge (pages 122–3)

7 Fish (pages 72–3)

8 Seated forward bend (pages 74–5)

9 Incline plane (pages 80–1)

10 King cobra (page 130)

11 Pigeon (pages 132–3)

12 Half spinal twist with bent legs (page 97)

13 Crow (pages 102–3)

14 Reverse triangle (page 107)

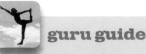

guru guide

• So that you are successful with the more challenging variations, keep your mind fully focused.

• Keep a diary of your practice to track your progress and remind you of how far you have come.

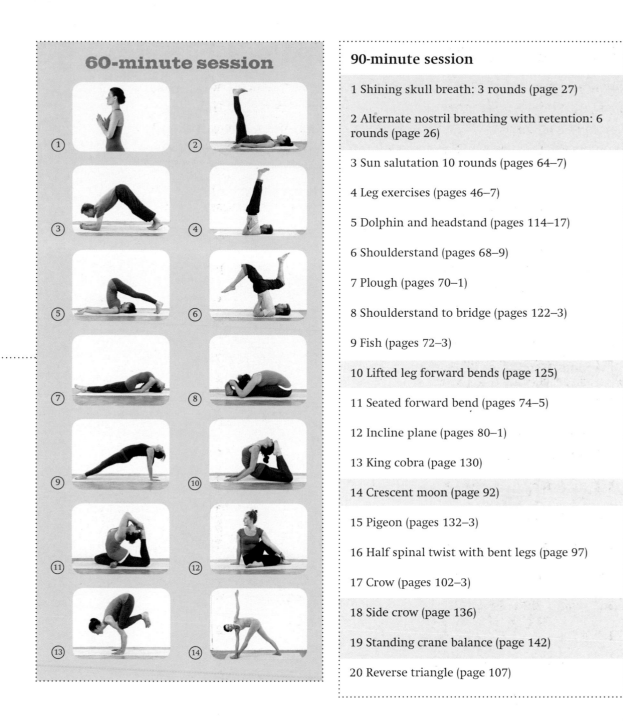

60-minute session

(1)
(2)
(3)
(4)
(5)
(6)
(7)
(8)
(9)
(10)
(11)
(12)
(13)
(14)

90-minute session

1 Shining skull breath: 3 rounds (page 27)

2 Alternate nostril breathing with retention: 6 rounds (page 26)

3 Sun salutation 10 rounds (pages 64–7)

4 Leg exercises (pages 46–7)

5 Dolphin and headstand (pages 114–17)

6 Shoulderstand (pages 68–9)

7 Plough (pages 70–1)

8 Shoulderstand to bridge (pages 122–3)

9 Fish (pages 72–3)

10 Lifted leg forward bends (page 125)

11 Seated forward bend (pages 74–5)

12 Incline plane (pages 80–1)

13 King cobra (page 130)

14 Crescent moon (page 92)

15 Pigeon (pages 132–3)

16 Half spinal twist with bent legs (page 97)

17 Crow (pages 102–3)

18 Side crow (page 136)

19 Standing crane balance (page 142)

20 Reverse triangle (page 107)

Visualizing the poses will help you achieve them; believe you can do them.

Advanced sessions 2

Advanced practice requires strength, flexibility and concentration, which you need to systematically build up to. Make sure you feel confident with the advanced sessions 1 before progressing to these ones. The variations included in these sessions give you confidence and strength of mind. Once you are in a pose, try to hold it as this gives tremendous mental and physical strength. Also aim to rest only briefly between each one.

The 45-minute session works on focus, balance and flexibility. **The 60-minute session** is a fully rounded practice, balancing the whole body and mind. **The 90-minute session** has a particular focus on back bends and balances. Start with 5 minutes relaxing in corpse pose (see page 31), then continue with your choice of routine and relax once more at the end in corpse pose for 10 minutes.

45-minute session

1 Sun salutation: 8 rounds (pages 64–7)

2 Dolphin and headstand (pages 114–17)

3 Shoulderstand (pages 68–9)

4 Plough (pages 70–1)

5 Shoulderstand to bridge (pages 122–3)

6 Fish (pages 72–3)

7 Balanced forward bend (page 125)

8 Incline plane (pages 80–1)

9 King cobra (page 130)

10 Half spinal twist with bent legs (page 97)

11 Head to toe pose (pages 108–9)

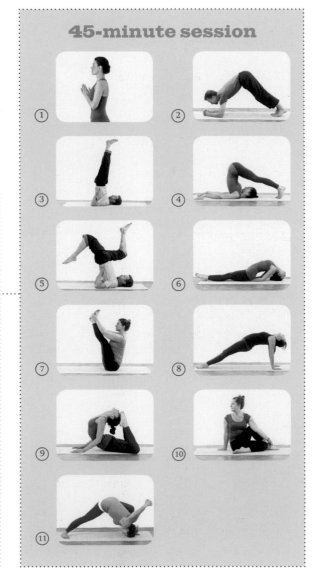

45-minute session

① ② ③ ④ ⑤ ⑥ ⑦ ⑧ ⑨ ⑩ ⑪

60-minute session

1 Shining skull breath: 3 rounds (page 27)

2 Alternate nostril breathing with retention: 10 rounds (page 26)

3 Sun salutation: 12 rounds (pages 64–7)

4 Dolphin and headstand (pages 114–17)

5 Shoulderstand (pages 68–9)

6 Plough (pages 70–1)

7 Shoulderstand to bridge (pages 122–3)

8 Fish (pages 72–3)

9 Balanced forward bend (page 125)

10 Incline plane (pages 80–1)

11 King cobra (page 130)

12 Full locust (page 131)

13 Half spinal twist with bent legs (page 97)

14 Extended leg side crow twist (page 137)

15 Hands to feet pose (pages 104–5)

16 Head to toe pose (pages 108–9)

guru guide

• Spend more time holding the poses and less time relaxing in-between.

• Make the practice a moving meditation and clearly set your intentions beforehand (see page 32).

• Spend more time on *pranayama* and introduce a meditation at the end to make you session longer.

90-minute session

1 Shining skull breath: 3 rounds (page 27)

2 Alternate nostril breathing with retention: 10 rounds (page 26)

3 Sun salutation: 12 rounds (pages 64–7)

4 Dolphin and headstand (pages 114–17)

5 Scorpion (pages 120–1)

6 Shoulderstand (pages 68–9)

7 Plough (pages 70–1)

8 Shoulderstand to bridge (pages 122–3)

9 Wheel (pages 126–7)

10 Fish (pages 72–3)

11 Tortoise (page 124)

12 Balanced forward bend (page 125)

13 Seated forward bend (pages 74–5)

14 Incline plane (pages 80–1)

15 King cobra (page 130)

16 Full locust (page 131)

17 Bow (pages 90–1)

18 Half spinal twist with bent legs (page 97)

19 Extended leg side crow twist (page 137)

20 Extended leg balancing twist (page 143)

21 Hands to feet pose (pages 104–5)

22 Head to toe pose (pages 108–9)

Relax at the end in corpse pose.

Energy booster

Give yourself a lift with some these yoga poses. If you are feeling sluggish or lethargic, roll out your mat and give yourself some natural energy. The poses are great to do before work, in your lunch break or at those times when you need a lift – just doing 15 minutes can make a huge difference.

Start with 5 minutes relaxing in corpse pose (see page 31), then continue with your choice of routine and relax once more at the end in corpse pose for 5 minutes.

30-minute session

1 Sun salutation: 6 rounds (pages 64–7)

2 Dynamic energizing squats (page 58)

3 Hands to feed pose (pages 104–5)

4 Triangle (page 106)

5 Warrior (page 110)

6 Cobra (pages 84–5)

7 Locust (pages 86–7)

8 Bow (pages 90–1)

9 Child's pose (page 30)

10 Tiptoe balancing twist (page 98)

11 Tree (pages 100–1)

15-minute session

1 Sun salutation: 4 rounds (pages 64–7)

2 Dynamic energizing squats (page 58)

3 Hands to feed pose (pages 104–5)

4 Triangle (page 106)

5 Warrior (page 110)

6 Tiptoe balancing twist (page 98)

7 Tree (pages 100–1)

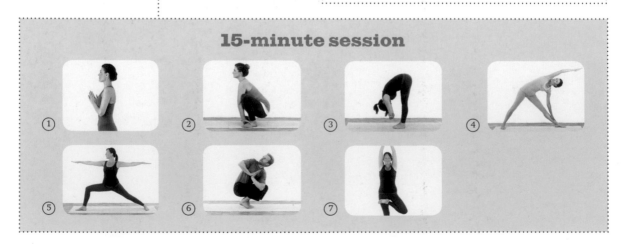

15-minute session

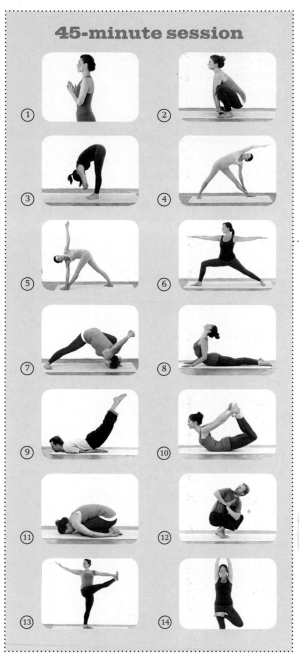

45-minute session

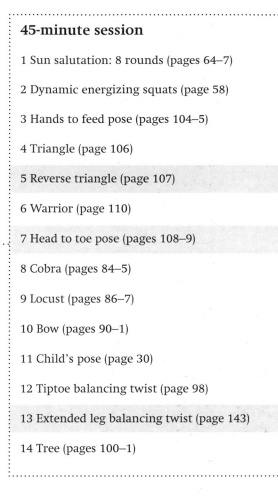

45-minute session

1 Sun salutation: 8 rounds (pages 64–7)

2 Dynamic energizing squats (page 58)

3 Hands to feed pose (pages 104–5)

4 Triangle (page 106)

5 Reverse triangle (page 107)

6 Warrior (page 110)

7 Head to toe pose (pages 108–9)

8 Cobra (pages 84–5)

9 Locust (pages 86–7)

10 Bow (pages 90–1)

11 Child's pose (page 30)

12 Tiptoe balancing twist (page 98)

13 Extended leg balancing twist (page 143)

14 Tree (pages 100–1)

guru guide

• Do all the poses given here as a flowing sequence and then relax.

• Practise sun salutation with the intention to wake up the fire and energy within you.

• To increase the cardiovascular effect of the sequence, make the movements dynamic and keep your arms raised as you move between the standing poses.

Roll out your mat and give yourself some natural energy.

Wind down

The poses in these sessions are chosen for their calming and relaxing effect, perfect for the evening and at those times when you simply need to be quite and calm. The sequences are nourishing and restorative. Do not rush them and rest between the postures if you need to.

Start with 5 minutes relaxing in corpse pose (page 31), then continue with your choice of routine and relax once more at the end in corpse pose for at least 10 minutes. You might also want to try some visualization (page 153).

15-minute session

1 Neck exercises (pages 38–9)

2 Shoulder rolls (pages 40–3)

3 Lying twist (page 49)

4 Sphinx (page 83)

5 Child's pose (page 30)

6 Thunderbolt (pages 94–5)

7 Alternate nostril breathing with or without retention: 6 rounds (page 26)

30-minute session

1 Neck exercises (pages 38–9)

2 Shoulder rolls (pages 40–3)

3 Bridge (page 48)

4 Lying twist (page 49)

5 Seated forward bend (pages 74–5)

6 Table top (page 81)

7 Sphinx (page 83)

8 Child's pose (page 30)

9 Thunderbolt (pages 94–5)

10 Alternate nostril breathing with or without retention: 6 rounds (page 26)

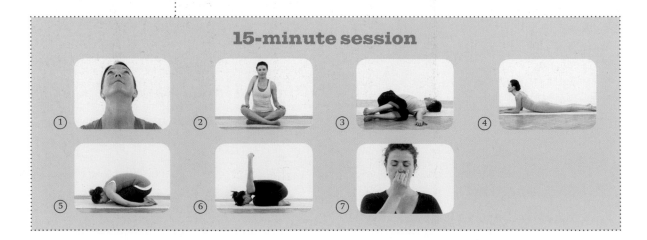

15-minute session

① ② ③ ④ ⑤ ⑥ ⑦

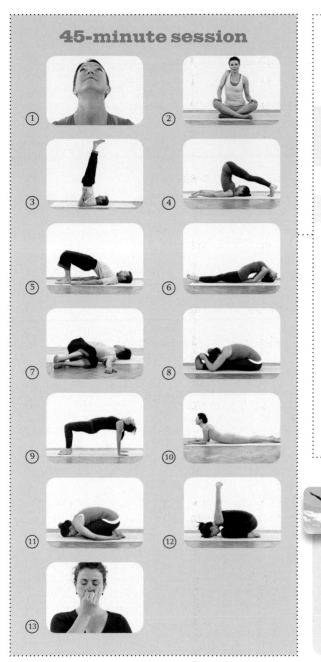

45-minute session

1 Neck exercises (pages 38–9)

2 Shoulder rolls (pages 40–3)

3 Shoulderstand (pages 68–9)

4 Plough (pages 70–1)

5 Bridge (page 48)

6 Fish (pages 72–3)

7 Lying twist (page 49)

8 Seated forward bend (pages 74–5)

9 Table top (page 81)

10 Sphinx (page 83)

11 Child's pose (page 30)

12 Thunderbolt (pages 94–5)

13 Alternate nostril breathing with or without retention: 8 rounds (page 26)

guru guide

• Practise with your eyes closed.

• Light a candle or burn some incense to create a relaxing atmosphere.

• Work slowly through the sequence and relax as much as you need to between poses.

These poses are perfect for the evening and at those times when you simply need to be calm.

Index

Credits

My Yoga Guru created for Octopus Publishing Group Ltd by:

Managing editor: Emma Callery
Designer: Alison Shackleton
Photographer: Nikki English

Models: Patrick Carpenter, Lila Conway, Liz Dillon,
Sarah Jenkins, Brigitte Suligoj
Hair and make-up: Anne-Marie Simak